# Diabetes

**YOUR QUESTIONS ANSWERED**

*Commissioning Editor*: Fiona Conn
*Project Development Manager*: Isobel Black
*Project Manager*: Frances Affleck
*Design Direction*: George Ajayi
*Illustration Manager*: Bruce Hogarth
*Illustrator*: Antbits

# Diabetes

# YOUR QUESTIONS ANSWERED

## Paul L Drury
MA MB BChir FRCP FRACP
Medical Director, Auckland Diabetes Centre,
Greenlane Clinical Centre,
Auckland;
Honorary Clinical Associate Professor in Medicine,
University of Auckland, Auckland, New Zealand

## Wendy Gatling
MB ChB DM FRCP
Consultant Physician, Department of Diabetes,
Poole Hospital NHS Trust,
Dorset, UK

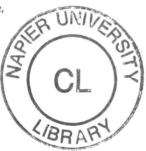

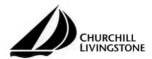

**CHURCHILL LIVINGSTONE**

EDINBURGH  LONDON  NEW YORK  OXFORD  PHILADELPHIA  ST LOUIS  SYDNEY  TORONTO  2005

CHURCHILL LIVINGSTONE
An imprint of Elsevier Limited

First published 2005

ISBN 0 4430 7389 9

**British Library Cataloguing in Publication Data**
A catalogue record for this book is available from the British Library

**Library of Congress Cataloging in Publication Data**
A catalog record for this book is available from the Library of Congress

**Notice**
Medical knowledge is constantly changing. Standard safety precautions must be followed, but as new research and clinical experience broaden our knowledge, changes in treatment and drug therapy may become necessary or appropriate. Readers are advised to check the most current product information provided by the manufacturer of each drug to be administered to verify the recommended dose, the method and duration of administration, and contraindications. It is the responsibility of the practitioner, relying on experience and knowledge of the patient, to determine dosages and the best treatment for each individual patient. Neither the Publisher nor the authors assume any liability for any injury and/or damage to persons or property arising from this publication.
*The Publisher*

The
publisher's
policy is to use
paper manufactured
from sustainable forests

Printed in China

# Contents

# Preface

Type 2 diabetes is increasing in prevalence across the world at epidemic rates. While the absolute prevalence varies widely between different countries and between ethnic groups, virtually all populations in the developed and developing world are showing dramatic increases in the burden of morbidity and mortality from diabetes and its complications.

In the UK, about 2–3% of the adult population now have diagnosed diabetes, while several immigrant populations (especially the South Asian and Afro-Caribbean) have much higher rates. In Australia and New Zealand perhaps 3–5% of the whole population now have diagnosed diabetes, with higher rates particularly in the Maori, Pacific Island, Aboriginal and Asian populations. Over 90% of patients with diabetes have type 2 disease (formerly called non-insulin dependent diabetes mellitus, NIDDM), even though the incidence of type 1 diabetes (insulin dependent diabetes mellitus, IDDM) is itself increasing, at least in younger age groups.

Beneath this epidemic lies an even greater problem with lesser degrees of glucose intolerance and insulin resistance (impaired glucose tolerance, impaired fasting glucose and the 'metabolic syndrome').

Until recently type 2 diabetes was the 'Cinderella' of endocrinology. The past 10–20 years have, however, seen dramatic developments in the treatment of diabetes and its complications. Technologies such as accurate blood glucose meters, insulin pens and a change in approach have enabled patients to achieve greater control over their disease. Major clinical trials have proved the value of strict glycaemic control in reducing the likelihood of complications, and of the effectiveness of many medical treatments in preventing both microvascular and macrovascular events. However, governments and health authorities have been slow to recognize the enormous morbidity, mortality and cost associated with inadequate intervention and prevention of complications. Increased resources and effective education of the health care professionals, especially those in primary care who predominantly care for people with diabetes, are critical to reducing the burden of diabetes on both patients and the health services. In addition, massive investment in public health measures is needed to reduce obesity and encourage healthier lifestyles.

This book aims to provide clear answers to a range of common questions often asked of specialists about diabetes. It is based on the best available evidence, but also includes practical consensus advice on common management issues where definitive data are not available. It is written primarily for GPs, but should also be valuable for the whole diabetes team in general practice and for all those professionals and students who come into frequent contact with these patients.

The structure of the book is intended to allow rapid access to the appropriate questions, but it is not a comprehensive textbook. Emphasis is placed on type 2 rather than type 1 disease, as this is both commoner and more often managed in general practice. Important areas where people with type 1 diabetes are managed differently are highlighted. References are largely recent and easily accessible (often on the Internet) rather than original data.

Many of the questions reflect those asked by patients. Diabetes is unique in requiring lifelong patient involvement in every aspect of their own management, and is frequently a joint learning experience for the individual, family and professional together. Thus we have also included both patient and professional sources of information and support.

Paul Drury
Wendy Gatling

# Acknowledgements

We owe a great deal to many past and present general practice colleagues for their questions. Similarly we wish to thank many present and past colleagues and teachers for their wisdom and advice, our patients for their insights, and our families for their forbearance. Any errors or mistakes are, however, our own.

# How to use this book

The *Your Questions Answered* series aims to meet the information needs of GPs and other primary care professionals who care for patients with chronic conditions. It is designed to help them work with patients and their families, providing effective, evidence-based care and management.

The books are in an accessible question and answer format, with detailed contents lists at the beginning of every chapter and a complete index to help find specific information.

## ICONS

Icons are used in the book to identify particular types of information:

 highlights information important to clinical practice

 highlights side-effect information.

 highlights case studies which illustrate or help to explain the answers given

## PATIENT QUESTIONS

At the end of relevant chapters there are sections of frequently asked patient questions, with easy-to-understand answers aimed at the non-medical reader. These questions are also listed at the end of the book.

# Background to diabetes

1

## DEFINITION AND CLASSIFICATION OF DIABETES

### 1.1    What is diabetes?

Diabetes (mellitus) is not a single entity but a group of conditions characterised by chronically raised plasma glucose concentrations. This glucose abnormality is due to an absolute or relative lack of insulin and has many causes, though commonest are 'type 2' and 'type 1' diabetes.

### 1.2    What controls insulin secretion?

In the healthy person, plasma glucose (PG) concentrations are controlled within a narrow range. The beta ($\beta$)-cells in the pancreatic islets of Langerhans continuously monitor the PG concentration; when glucose levels start to rise, most usually after a meal, insulin is secreted into the pancreatic circulation, which drains into the portal vein. Insulin passes to the liver before moving into the systemic circulation. Within the liver, insulin increases glucose uptake and storage as glycogen. It is also the key to glucose uptake peripherally, particularly in muscle. Pancreatic insulin secretion thus lowers PG concentration by increasing both storage and peripheral glucose uptake.

As glucose levels fall, the pancreas switches off insulin secretion. If PG falls below about 4 mmol/l, the alpha ($\alpha$)-cells of the pancreas secrete glucagon, which stimulates hepatic glucose production by breakdown of glycogen. This is an important part of the response to hypoglycaemia, though not the total story.

### 1.3    What is 'normal' blood glucose?

In healthy humans, fasting PG is closely regulated and overnight fasting or pre-prandial PG levels are usually between 3.8 and 5.5 mmol/l. PG may fall on prolonged (24 hours or greater) fasting, especially in women, but gluconeogenesis prevents significant hypoglycaemia occurring. Plasma glucose levels increase to 5–7 mmol/l around 30–90 minutes after a meal, before falling rapidly to normal. A greater and faster increase in PG concentration occurs following an oral glucose tolerance test (OGTT) or similar glycaemic challenge (e.g. a large drink of 'Coke'). In both instances, PG levels will fall to baseline levels within 2–3 hours of the meal, and a daytime profile would show predominantly basal PGs of around 4–5 mmol/l.

Random plasma glucose values above 7 mmol/l are suspicious of some degree of glucose intolerance (unless sampled at peak time after an unusual glucose challenge), while fasting levels above 5.5 mmol/l may indicate glucose intolerance or even diabetes.

> Plasma, whole blood and capillary glucoses are slightly different. Venous whole blood glucose (BG) is generally about 0.5–1.0 mmol/l lower than venous plasma values or capillary whole blood. It is important to be clear which is being reported as the ranges for diagnosis differ.

## 1.4 What are the different types of diabetes?

There are several types of diabetes (*Box 1.1*), most commonly type 1 and type 2 diabetes. This book deals principally with type 2 and it is important to be aware of the differences in pathophysiology.

*Type 1 diabetes*

Type 1 diabetes is due to the destruction of the pancreatic islet cells, usually but not always autoimmune in nature. It is characterised by a relatively

---

**BOX 1.1  Aetiological classification of disorders of glucose control**

■ Type 1 (beta-cell destruction, usually leading to absolute insulin deficiency)
  — autoimmune
  — idiopathic
■ Type 2 (may range from predominantly insulin resistance with relative insulin deficiency to a predominantly secretory defect with or without insulin resistance)
■ Other specific types
  — genetic defects of beta-cell function (e.g. chromosome 7, chromosome 20, HNF-4-alpha (MODY 1), glucokinase (MODY 2), HNF-1-alpha (MODY 3))
  — genetic defects in insulin secretion
  — diseases of the exocrine pancreas (e.g. pancreatitis, cystic fibrosis, haemochromatosis, pancreatectomy)
  — endocrine causes (e.g. Cushing's syndrome, acromegaly)
  — drug- or chemical-induced (e.g. steroids)
  — infections (e.g. congenital rubella, cytomegalovirus)
  — uncommon forms of immune-mediated diabetes
  — other genetic syndromes sometimes associated with diabetes (e.g. Down's syndrome, myotonic dystrophy)
■ Gestational diabetes

Adapted from Alberti et al.[3] HNF, hepatic nuclear factor; MODY, maturity onset diabetes of the young.

short history of typical symptoms – severe insulin deficiency results in marked hyperglycaemia and eventually ketosis due to fat breakdown. Without insulin, these patients eventually develop life-threatening diabetic ketoacidosis. While commoner in young people, it can occur at any age.

### Type 2 diabetes

Type 2 diabetes has a more insidious onset, often asymptomatic and unrecognised for many years. Patients still produce some insulin but insufficient to adequately control PG levels within the narrow normal range. It is usually coupled with some degree of insulin 'resistance', requiring more insulin than normal in order to lower glucose levels.

## 1.5    What is the difference between type 1 and type 2 diabetes?

Type 1 diabetes is essentially absence of significant insulin secretion from the pancreas, leading to a classical hormone deficiency syndrome eventually leading to total insulin deficiency and, if untreated, to ketoacidosis. As an approximation, these patients would be secreting less than 10% of normal insulin when diagnosed and virtually none after 5 years of diabetes.

In contrast, type 2 diabetes involves a milder degree of insulin deficiency usually with a variable amount of insulin resistance (reduced insulin sensitivity). There must be at least some degree of insulin deficiency – resistance alone is not enough.

Both forms have a prodromal phase where there is evidence of the disease process at work – largely immunological in type 1 disease and biochemical in type 2 – when PG levels are little, if at all, altered and so patients are asymptomatic. Once PG concentrations are significantly raised, people with type 1 diabetes require insulin treatment within a short period. Initially, those with type 2 diabetes can usually be treated with dietary/lifestyle measures and oral hypoglycaemic agents.[1] Later, when insulin secretion is reduced further, exogenous insulin is often required to control PG levels adequately. The need for insulin treatment does not, however, change type 2 into type 1 diabetes, a common misunderstanding.

Less common types of diabetes are the secondary causes, including those caused by pancreatic and endocrine disease, genetic syndromes and drug-induced diabetes (*see Box 1.1*). Exhaustive lists are given in the American Diabetes Association and World Health Organization classifications.[2–4]

## HOW TO DIAGNOSE DIABETES

### 1.6 Exactly how is diabetes now diagnosed?

Diabetes can only be diagnosed on the basis of a laboratory glucose measurement. The small meters used by patients and professionals to monitor diabetes, while increasingly accurate, are not reliable enough for a final diagnosis of diabetes. After all, the diagnosis is for life and has a major impact on the patient's lifestyle, so must be undertaken with appropriate care.

The WHO has formalised the diagnostic criteria for diabetes (*Table 1.1*). These are set to distinguish those people who have glucose levels that make them at risk of microvascular diabetes complications (e.g. retinopathy, nephropathy and neuropathy). In the population, PG concentrations demonstrate a range just like many other biological variables such as height, weight, BP, etc. The continuous nature of the distribution of PG concentrations inevitably means that, when a line is drawn to mark the diagnostic cut-off point, some people will fall either just above or just below the line. Many of those just below will have impaired glucose tolerance (IGT) or impaired fasting glucose (IFG).[5]

**TABLE 1.1 World Health Organization diagnostic criteria for diabetes**[2,3]

| | Plasma glucose concentration | |
| | mmol/l | mg/dl |
| --- | --- | --- |
| **Diabetes mellitus** | | |
| Fasting | ≥ 7.0 | ≥ 126 |
| *or* | | |
| 2-hour post glucose load | ≥ 11.1 | ≥ 200 |
| *or both* | | |
| **Impaired glucose tolerance** | | |
| Fasting | < 7.0 | < 126 |
| *and* | | |
| 2-hour post glucose load | ≥ 7.8 and <11.1 | ≥ 140 and < 200 |
| **Impaired fasting glycaemia\*** | | |
| Fasting | ≥ 6.1 and < 7.0 | ≥ 110 and < 126 |
| 2 hour | < 7.8 | < 140 |

\* An oral glucose tolerance test should normally be undertaken to exclude diabetes. Figures for whole blood capillary and whole blood venous levels are lower and are given in full in references 3 and 24. Meter glucose levels should not be used for diagnosis.

## 1.7    Which is the best blood sample to diagnose diabetes?

A laboratory glucose concentration is required to diagnose both type 2 and type 1 diabetes, so this test is obligatory: a meter reading is not sufficient. The diagnostic criteria are based on either a raised fasting or a raised 2-hour level. Blood/plasma glucose varies quite widely, rising after meals, making interpretation difficult. For this reason, the fasting PG has been widely used in diagnosing diabetes and all authorities agree that a fasting PG level of 7.0 mmol/l or more is diagnostic, though a confirmatory sample on a separate occasion is essential where there are no clear symptoms (*see Case vignettes 1.1–1.3*).

However, a fasting glucose may not be the most sensitive first-line test. Some patients whose fasting PG is below 7.0 mmol/l will have diabetes as defined by a 2-hour glucose tolerance test value of 11.1 mmol/l or more. The 2-hour level is more sensitive and specific for risk of diabetic complications and for the increased risk of cardiovascular disease.

The intermediate 2-hour post-glucose level between diabetes (≥ 11.1 mmol/l) and normal (< 7.8 mmol/l) is termed 'impaired glucose tolerance'.

Some people have a raised fasting glucose between 6.0 and 6.9 mmol/l but with a normal 2-hour glucose on OGTT. This is called 'impaired fasting glucose or glycaemia' – such people have a higher risk of cardiovascular disease than the normal population but not as high as those with 'impaired glucose tolerance' or diabetes itself. Patients with IGT or IFG are not at risk of 'diabetic' microvascular complications.

In practice, if a patient presents with typical symptoms of diabetes and significant glycosuria, a random laboratory PG ≥ 11.1 mmol/l is diagnostic for diabetes and will usually clinch the diagnosis. In a patient with no obvious symptoms, a laboratory PG taken 2 hours after a main meal is a good first-line test. In some cases (e.g. when monitoring lipid profiles at the same time), a fasting glucose will be undertaken. A fasting PG ≥ 7.0 mmol/l is diagnostic but if it falls in the range of 5.5–6.9 mmol/l, a full OGTT should be requested. There are currently some moves to lower the IFG threshold to 5.6 mmol/l.

Current action for different fasting PG levels should be:

- ≥ 7.0 mmol/l → diabetes present if confirmed on second sample
- 6.1–6.9 mmol/l → needs OGTT, may be IGT or IFG
- 5.5–6.0 mmol/l → diabetes or IGT unlikely but possible, needs OGTT
- <5.5 mmol/l → diabetes extremely unlikely – no action needed.

An abnormal HbA1c means diabetes is extremely likely, but is not part of the current diagnostic criteria. One study comparing HbA1c with an OGTT found that only 2 of 178 people (<2%) with an abnormal HbA1c did not have diabetes, but 64 (36%) diagnosed with diabetes on the OGTT had a normal HbA1c.

### CASE VIGNETTE 1.1

An Indian lady, aged 56 years, with long-standing hypertension is found to have 1% glycosuria at her regular check. Fasting plasma glucose is 7.5 mmol/l. Does she have diabetes?

*Comment*

She probably has diabetes as the fasting PG is above the diagnostic criteria (≥7.0 mmol/l). According to the WHO diagnostic criteria, diabetes can be diagnosed on the basis of a single abnormal laboratory PG concentration in the presence of typical symptoms. If she is asymptomatic, then a further diagnostic PG is required. A repeat fasting PG ≥7.0 mmol/l would confirm this, otherwise a glucose tolerance test is required.

### CASE VIGNETTE 1.2

A previously fit 67-year-old man now complains of non-specific tiredness. A random PG is 10.1 mmol/l, and a subsequent OGTT showed a fasting PG of 7.2 mmol/l and 2-hour level of 9.7 mmol/l. Does he have diabetes?

*Comment*

The random PG is not diagnostic for diabetes, being less than the critical level of 11.1 mmol/l. Thus an OGTT was requested. The fasting PG is above 7.0 mmol/l but the 2-hour glucose is below the diagnostic cut-off. The WHO diagnostic criteria require *either* the fasting *or* the 2-hour PG to be above the cut-off to make a diagnosis but also state that, in the absence of specific symptoms, diagnostic PG levels on two occasions are required to make the diagnosis. This patient requires a repeat test undertaken and a fasting PG test will probably confirm the diagnosis. If a diagnosis of diabetes is not confirmed, he should have regular repeat checks, perhaps every 6–12 months.

### CASE VIGNETTE 1.3

This sprightly 72-year-old lady, treated with thyroxine 0.1 mg daily for primary hypothyroidism, now complains of losing 5 kg of weight in the last 2 months and is very thirsty. Her current weight is 58 kg with a BMI of 22.1 kg/m². What is the most likely diagnosis?

*Comment*

She probably has type 1 diabetes. She is lean, markedly symptomatic and has lost a significant amount of weight. As she already has another autoimmune disease (primary hypothyroidism), a high index of suspicion is necessary. In a highly symptomatic patient, a random laboratory PG is usually over 11 mmol/l and is thus adequate to make the diagnosis of diabetes. A positive urine ketone test may confirm your suspicion of insulin deficiency – alternatively a positive glutamic acid dehydrogenase (GAD) antibody test will strengthen the case for type 1 diabetes. In some instances, however, it is necessary to start insulin treatment on clinical grounds; these are good cases to land on your local specialist!

## 1.8 Is urine testing still a good way to detect diabetes?

The presence of glycosuria is suggestive of diabetes but its absence does not exclude diabetes. In most people, the normal renal threshold for glucose is 10 mmol/l; when PG exceeds this, some glycosuria is found. In people with diabetes (e.g. when fasting), PG may be abnormal but still below 10 mmol/l. Thus a first morning urine sample is an insensitive sample to detect diabetes.

The renal threshold for glucose in some people is considerably lower than 10 mmol/l so that glycosuria is found at normal PG concentrations. For instance, the renal threshold is lower during pregnancy, particularly in the second and third trimesters. In others, the renal threshold is above 10 mmol/l, often in the elderly. With all these problems, urine testing is not a good screening test. That said, glycosuria found on a routine examination should always be followed up.

## 1.9 How common is undiagnosed diabetes or glucose intolerance in the population?

> Studies in many populations have shown undiagnosed diabetes to be roughly as common as diagnosed cases, while variable numbers also have IGT or IFG. Accurate figures are problematical because the criteria for IGT and IFG have changed over the years. The AUSDIAB study is a recent example showing doubling of the prevalence of diabetes in Australia over the past 20 years (from 3.4 to 7.2%), while undiagnosed diabetes remains as common as those with definite diabetes.[6]

## 1.10 Is systematic screening for type 2 diabetes justified?

Current evidence is incomplete for population screening for diabetes.

It is well recognised that type 2 diabetes has an insidious onset: many patients are not diagnosed until years of chronic hyperglycaemia have elapsed. Consequently, it is not uncommon to find evidence of long-term complications at the time of diagnosis; indeed, symptoms of a complication may be the reason for presentation rather than hyperglycaemia! Many studies in both type 1 and type 2 diabetes have shown that poor glycaemic control is related to a higher risk of long-term complications (*see Ch. 2*). Thus, screening for diabetes would intrinsically seem a good idea – identifying the condition before symptoms and complications develop – but scientific proof of benefit and cost-effectiveness is still lacking.[7-9] To date, no trial has shown that early identification of diabetes through screening leads to a reduction in long-term complications.

The approach suggested is to screen high-risk individuals opportunistically rather than the whole population (*Box 1.2*). Those at risk include people thought to have the 'metabolic syndrome'. The National Service Framework for Diabetes for England and Wales, published in 2002,[10] has included the necessity of early identification of diabetes and will probably lead to the establishment of a screening programme in primary care.

---

**BOX 1.2  People at high risk of developing diabetes**

■ Those with:
  — a family history of type 2 diabetes
  — a previous history of gestational diabetes
  — obesity (especially central)
  — metabolic syndrome
  — hypertension
  — gout
  — ischaemic heart disease
  — cerebrovascular disease
  — peripheral vascular disease
  — recurrent skin infections
■ People using drugs including steroids and high-dose thiazide diuretics

---

### 1.11  Is there such a thing as 'mild' diabetes?

No. Present evidence suggests that all patients with diabetes have a significant risk of microvascular disease. This is much higher with poor glycaemic control than with good control, but even at HbA1c levels regarded as 'excellent' (6.0–6.5%) there are still some risks of retinopathy, nephropathy and neuropathy.

For macrovascular disease, the answer is even clearer: a substantially increased risk of coronary, cerebrovascular and peripheral vascular disease is present even before the stage of diabetes is reached. Indeed, patients with IGT or metabolic syndrome *who do not have diabetes* show two- to three-fold increases in cardiovascular morbidity.

To reassure patients that their disease is 'mild' is neither true nor helpful, as it frequently produces or reinforces denial of the need for energetic treatment and supervision.

---

## THE METABOLIC SYNDROME AND OTHER ABNORMALITIES OF GLUCOSE TOLERACE

---

### 1.12  What is the 'metabolic syndrome'?

This term, coined about 15 years ago by Gerald Reaven and also known as 'Syndrome X', has grown in importance as the global epidemic of obesity and diabetes has become apparent. People with the combination of hypertension, central obesity, dyslipidaemia and hyperglycaemia are said to have the 'metabolic syndrome'. These people are at high risk of developing macrovascular disease. Insulin resistance is believed to be a key component of the syndrome and to a number of metabolically unfavourable changes. All these factors have adverse cardiovascular associations, and many are closely inter-related.

However, there is no easy test for the metabolic syndrome or a simple measure of insulin resistance. The WHO, the National Cholesterol Education Program in the US (NCEP-ATP III) and the European Group of Insulin Resistance have all produced slightly different recommended criteria, though each involves counting up characteristics of a syndrome that is necessarily continuous. Thus the WHO definition requires a degree of glucose intolerance but NCEP does not. Many authorities consider that any such cut-off figures – be they for obesity, waist circumference, lipid levels or microalbuminuria – are artificial. The various components of the metabolic syndrome are listed with their cardiovascular relevance in *Box 1.3*.[11–14]

## 1.13 How common is the metabolic syndrome?

Extremely common, even more so than diabetes. It would appear that 25% of all US adults now meet the NCEP criteria; this has increased dramatically over the past 10 years.

---

**BOX 1.3 Definitions and features of the metabolic syndrome**

**Definition: World Health Organization**
- Glucose intolerance, impaired glucose tolerance or diabetes, and/or insulin resistance with two or more of the following:
  — raised arterial pressure $\geq$160/90 mmHg
  — raised plasma triglyceride ($\geq$1.7 mmol/l (150 mg/dl) and/or low HDL cholesterol (<0.9 mmol/l (35 mg/dl) for men and <1 mmol/l (39 mg/dl) for women)
  — central obesity (males: waist to hip ratio >0.90; females: waist to hip ratio >0.85) and/or BMI >30 kg/m$^2$
  — microalbuminuria (urinary albumin excretion rate $\geq$20 mcg/min or albumin:creatinine ratio $\geq$20 mg/g)

**Definition: National Cholesterol Education Program: Adult treatment panel (ATP III)**
- Any three of the following:
  — waist girth >102 cm (40 ins) in men or >88 cm (35 ins) in women
  — triglycerides $\geq$1.7 mmol/l (150 mg/dl)
  — HDL cholesterol <1.0 mmol/l in men or <1.3 mmol/l in women (40 mg/dl and 50 mg/dl, respectively)
  — blood pressure $\geq$130 mmHg systolic or $\geq$85 mmHg diastolic
  — fasting glucose $\geq$6.1 mmol/l (110 mg/dl)

---

**BOX 1.3** (*Cont'd*) **Definitions and features of the metabolic syndrome**

**Clinical features**

■ Insulin resistance
■ Central (abdominal) obesity
■ Dyslipidaemia
■ Increased blood pressure
■ Microalbuminuria
■ Other manifestations:
— gout/hyperuricaemia
— coagulation disorders
— increased plasminogen activator inhibitor 1
— non-alcoholic fatty liver disease

See references 11, 25, 26.

---

People identified as having metabolic syndrome should be screened regularly for diabetes, and will also need cardiovascular risk factor assessment and intervention.

## 1.14 Is type 2 diabetes related to the metabolic syndrome?

Yes. Glucose intolerance of all degrees is one component of the metabolic syndrome in which insulin resistance is thought to be a primary abnormality (*Fig. 1.1*). In the developed world, where obesity is common, most people with type 2 diabetes have several features of the metabolic syndrome, suggesting a predominantly insulin-resistant problem. In contrast, populations where obesity is less common tend to have more type 2 diabetes related to insulin deficiency.

## 1.15 What exactly is 'insulin resistance'?

This term – equally well described as loss of normal insulin sensitivity – implies that one or more tissues do not respond normally to insulin: the most important tissues are liver, muscle and fat cells. Resistance may take the form of decreased uptake of glucose into the cell, or reduced inhibition of a cellular function by insulin. Only very rarely is there a specific cause such as an abnormality of the insulin receptor itself or the insulin molecule.

Insulin resistance inevitably leads to increased insulin secretion in an attempt to overcome the resistance. With healthy pancreatic beta-cells, this results in increased insulin secretion which initially maintains normal cellular metabolism. If the beta-cells are damaged, they fail to maintain this increased secretion. The speed of failure may depend on the individual's susceptibility related to both genetic and environmental factors. The

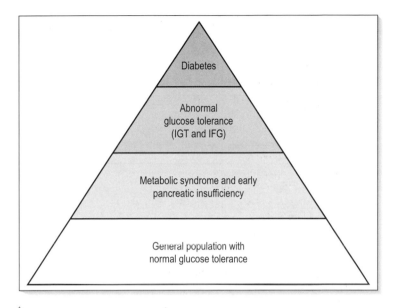

▲

**Fig. 1.1** The 'iceberg' of glucose intolerance and metabolic syndrome in a population.

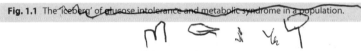

progressive decline in beta-cell function leads to an increasing PG concentration – this is thought by some to be 'toxic' to the beta-cells, speeding up their death.

## 1.16 What should be done when impaired glucose tolerance or impaired fasting glycaemia is found?

People with IGT or IFG do not have diabetes and will not develop the *microvascular* complications of diabetes. However, they have a substantially increased risk of developing *macrovascular* disease (e.g. coronary artery disease, stroke and peripheral arterial disease).[15]

The natural history of IGT varies between the populations studied. In one Caucasian population studied for 10 years, 15% developed type 2 diabetes, a significant number remained with IGT and just over half returned to normal glucose tolerance.[16] Those with initial fasting PG ≥5.5 mmol/l seem to be at highest risk of developing diabetes – some recent trials showed much higher conversion rates over shorter periods although these were mainly US studies.[1,17,18]

Several recent randomised trials including Finnish and Chinese studies, the Diabetes Prevention Program (DPP)[1] and XENDOS[19] have shown that weight loss and regular exercise can reduce the incidence of diabetes by nearly 60%. The DPP also used metformin, and STOP-NIDDM[20] used acarbose while the XENDOS study also used orlistat to help achieve significant weight loss.

The management strategy for people with IGT should include:

- screen and treat cardiovascular risk factors – hypertension, smoking, hyperlipidaemia
- review drug therapy – stop or reduce dose of thiazide diuretics, beta-blockers and steroids
- weight-reducing diet with low sugar, low fat intake (aim for loss of at least 7% of initial body weight)
- promote physical activity (at least 150 minutes per week)
- annual fasting glucose or OGTT to detect progression to diabetes.

IFG is a recently introduced category and less is known about the long-term outcome. Present data suggest that those with IFG are still at higher risk of developing diabetes and macrovascular disease, but less so than for IGT. A simplistic explanation is that the IGT group has more insulin resistance while the IFG group has less insulin secretion and suppression of hepatic glucose output.[5]

## THE PREVENTION OF DIABETES

### 1.17 Can type 2 diabetes be prevented?

This is a difficult question. For the individual patient who is not obese, but has a strong family history of diabetes presenting in middle age or earlier, it is doubtful if anything can currently be done to prevent pancreatic failure as the mechanisms leading to beta-cell failure are not clear. On the other hand, in the obese patient with IGT, weight loss combined with an exercise programme can substantially reduce progression to diabetes, at least over the medium term.

The DPP randomised 3234 non-diabetic people aged ≥ 25 years and BMI ≥ 24 kg/m$^2$ with a fasting PG of 5.3–6.9 mmol/l and 2 hours after 75 g OGTT had a PG of 7.8–11.0 mmol/l to one of three intervention arms.[1] Standard lifestyle intervention included written information and an annual individual session emphasising a healthy lifestyle plus a placebo tablet twice daily. The same standard lifestyle intervention was combined with metformin 850 mg tablet twice daily in the second arm. The third arm was an intensive lifestyle modification with goals to achieve and maintain at least 7% weight reduction through a low calorie, low fat diet combined with physical activity of moderate intensity for at least 150 minutes per week achieved through individual sessions of a 16-lesson curriculum in the first 6 months and then monthly individual or group sessions. Follow-up was for a mean of 2.8 years. In the intensive arm, 50% achieved 7% weight reduction at

24 weeks with 38% maintaining 7% weight reduction at the end of the study. The incidence of diabetes was 11.0, 7.8 and 4.8 cases per 100 person-years in the placebo, metformin and intensive lifestyle modification groups, respectively. The intensive lifestyle modification programme reduced the incidence of diabetes by 58% and metformin by 31% as compared to placebo (*Fig. 1.2*). Intensive lifestyle was significantly more effective than metformin.

Two other randomised controlled studies of people with IGT from Finland and China have demonstrated a 55–60% reduction in progression to type 2 diabetes with lifestyle modification.[17,18] In addition, the Finnish group demonstrated that subjects in both the intervention and control groups who achieved most lifestyle change virtually prevented progression to diabetes, whilst those who did not modify lifestyles had little if any protection. However, it must be emphasized that these short-term studies (3–5 years), all performed in people with IGT, required considerable resources and have so far only shown *delay* rather than permanent prevention.

It has also been shown that women with previous gestational diabetes randomised to the thiazolidinedione, troglitazone, demonstrated a significant reduction in incidence of diabetes compared with placebo.

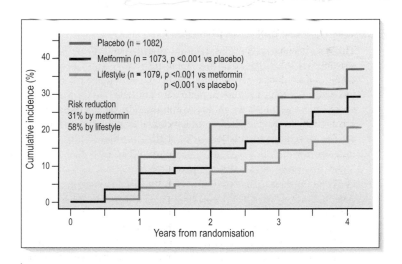

**Fig. 1.2** Diabetes Prevention Programme: cumulative incidence of diabetes in placebo, metformin and lifestyle intervention groups. (From Diabetes Prevention Program Research Group.[1] Copyright © 2002 Massachusetts Medical Society. All rights reserved.)

Troglitazone has now been withdrawn due to liver side effects but studies with rosiglitazone and pioglitazone are underway.

Unfortunately, these interventions were neither simple nor affordable and have not been studied in a general population where they may be even less practicable and cost-effective.

### 1.18  Can type 1 diabetes be prevented, and should we be screening for it?

Unfortunately the answer remains no. While there are clear ways of identifying individuals at high risk of type 1 diabetes from their genetic (human leucocyte antigen, HLA) markers and pancreatic-related autoantibodies, all trials of potentially protective agents including nicotinamide and oral/subcutaneous insulin have so far been negative. With the aid of insulin secretory tests such as the intravenous glucose tolerance test, it is possible to follow the degree of destruction of beta-cells but, as yet, no intervention has been shown to halt this destructive process. In the absence of any effective intervention there is no point in screening.

Possible exceptions could be made where the results would affect a major decision, for example a sibling of a person with type 1 diabetes thinking of becoming an airline pilot.

## THE PATHOPHYSIOLOGY AND AETIOLOGY OF DIABETES

### 1.19  What are the mechanisms leading to diabetes?

*Question 1.2* discussed the control of PG concentrations over a narrow range by pancreatic beta-cell glucose sensing and insulin secretion. In response to the PG concentration rising, the immediate (first-phase) release of insulin reaches a peak within a few minutes and enhances glucose uptake within minutes. In the healthy person, this substantially limits the post-prandial rise in PG. Within approximately 2 hours, PG returns to normal fasting levels. Oral feeding also produces gut hormone release, which enhances the first-phase insulin release compared with that obtained by an equal amount of intravenous glucose.

Type 1 diabetes develops gradually and the first-phase insulin secretion is progressively reduced as the autoimmune process damages the islet cells. Normally, there is only a small second phase of insulin secretion as PG rapidly returns to normal and there is no continued stimulus to insulin secretion. Second-phase insulin secretion is thought to result from increased insulin synthesis within the beta-cell, as opposed to immediate release of pre-formed insulin granules that characterises the first-phase response. When the first-phase response is reduced or absent, PG rises and provides a continuing stimulus to insulin synthesis and subsequent secretion in order to maintain fasting glucose. It is generally reckoned that

80–90% of insulin secretory capacity must be lost in type 1 diabetes before there is any noticeable change in glucose metabolism.

In type 2 diabetes, there is always a decrease in insulin secretion, but it is associated with a variable degree of insulin resistance. Given normal insulin secretion, insulin resistance alone (no matter how severe) is unlikely to produce diabetes, as there is substantial spare secretory capacity within the pancreatic beta-cells.

The precise pathogenesis of type 2 diabetes remains unknown, but in most instances is a very insidious process. Natural history studies have shown that insulin secretion first increases in an attempt to overcome the resistance and it is only when the deficiency becomes severe enough that the increased insulin secretion fails to compensate for the insulin resistance (*Fig. 1.3*). In some respects, this is like a 'Starling curve' of the pancreas.

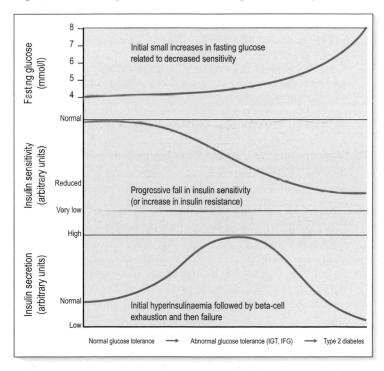

**Fig. 1.3** Graphic showing the usual progression from normal glucose tolerance to diabetes. Initially decreased insulin sensitivity leads to increased secretion, then to beta-cell exhaustion. Changes in glucose tolerance and particularly fasting glucose are relatively late.

With time, insulin secretion declines further and hyperglycaemia becomes progressively more severe, eventually leading to symptomatic diabetes. The process is much longer than the decline in pancreatic function seen in type 1 diabetes, and patients frequently remain undiagnosed for many years. Several studies relating the prevalence of retinopathy in different groups to the duration of diagnosed diabetes have suggested that this prodromal period of undiagnosed diabetes may be as long as 5–15 years (*see Q. 2.1* and *Fig. 2.2*).

---

### 1.20  How much genetic component is there to type 2 diabetes?

Only a few patients with type 2 diabetes have a single defined genetic abnormality such as maturity onset diabetes of the young (MODY) syndromes. There are also a large number of extremely rare specific genetic syndromes, but these make up only a tiny proportion of all those with type 2 diabetes. The commonest form, MODY 3, is due to a mutation in a hepatic nuclear factor, HNF-1alpha.

In the remainder of patients no single or multiple gene abnormalities have been identified to date, though there are clear familial elements in its distribution suggesting a significant genetic component. For example, identical twins with type 2 diabetes are almost always concordant (both twins having diabetes, and usually developing at similar ages), which is far from the situation in type 1 diabetes where less than 50% are concordant. Similarly, many families can trace a high prevalence of diabetes through several generations, though there is no clear pattern of a specific form of inheritance.

---

### 1.21  What is known about the genetic and familial inheritance of type 1 diabetes?

With type 1 diabetes, the *susceptibility* to the disease is inherited, not the disease itself. This has best been shown by HLA typing where the high-risk types (DR3 and DR4) show increased susceptibility. The majority of individuals with these high-risk genotypes will not develop type 1 diabetes, but the relative risk of such a genotype becoming diabetic is many times higher than for an individual of a low-risk genotype. An environmental agent, at present unidentified, triggers the autoimmune process, which is accompanied by the presence of autoimmune markers such as islet-cell, GAD and insulin antibodies. In most studies in European populations, only 10% of those with type 1 diabetes have a first-degree relative with the disease, leaving 90% occurring as 'sporadic' cases. Consequently only population screening would be effective, and that only if effective preventative methods have been found (*see Q. 1.18*).

## 1.22 How strong is the link between type 2 diabetes and obesity?

Extremely powerful. Data from the US Nurses Health Study and other sources indicate a positive and exponential relationship between obesity and future risk of diabetes, as shown in *Figure 1.4*. Thus, a woman with a BMI of 30 kg/m² has roughly 30 times the risk of developing diabetes compared with someone of BMI 22 kg/m², while an individual with a BMI ≥ 35 kg/m² has a 90-fold higher risk.[21] That said, the AUSDIAB study showed increases in prevalence over recent years even at similar levels of BMI.[6]

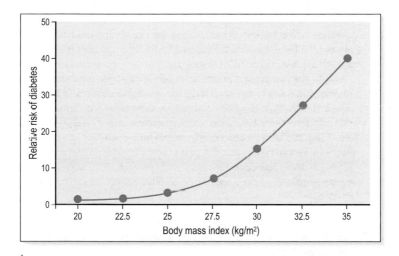

**Fig. 1.4** The relationship between obesity and subsequent relative risk of diabetes. Note the exponential rise with severe degrees of overweight.

## THE EPIDEMIOLOGY OF DIABETES

## 1.23 How common is type 2 diabetes in the UK?

Currently, about 2.5–3% of the UK adult population has diagnosed type 2 diabetes. The prevalence varies widely between countries and ethnic groups, being uncommon in childhood and adolescence. As people get older, diabetes becomes increasingly common with approximately 10% of European populations aged over 70 having diagnosed type 2 diabetes.

Population studies in many countries have also shown a large number of people with undiagnosed diabetes, generally equivalent in number to those with the diagnosed condition.

### 1.24 How much does the prevalence of type 2 diabetes vary with age, sex and ethnicity?

Age and ethnicity are the most important factors in determining the prevalence of type 2 diabetes. All populations studied show a considerable increase in diabetes prevalence with increasing age. In many countries, there is little difference in the prevalence between men and women, but in some the male prevalence is slightly greater. For example, in 1996 the prevalence of diagnosed diabetes was significantly higher in men than in women, 2.1% versus 1.6%, in the Poole (UK) Diabetes Study[22] due to a higher incidence in men: 2.3 new cases per 1000 compared to 1.7 in women.

Type 2 diabetes is commoner amongst non-European ethnic groups. In the UK, those of Afro-Caribbean and Indo-Asian origin have roughly three to four times more diabetes than in the European population. In New Zealand and Australia, it is similarly commoner in Maori, Aboriginal, Pacific Island and both South and East Asian groups than in Europeans (*Fig. 1.5*). Not only do all these populations have a significantly higher

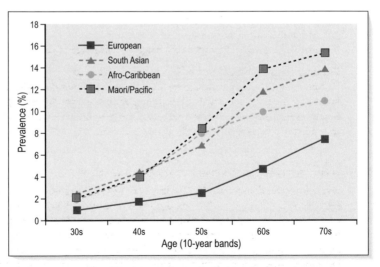

▲

**Fig. 1.5** The effect of age and different ethnicities on diabetes prevalence. Data from multiple sources during 1990s. Note that diabetes occurs substantially earlier in non-European groups.

prevalence of diabetes, but it also develops at a younger age, perhaps 7–10 years earlier. These populations also tend to have even more people with undiagnosed diabetes and IGT/IGF than European populations.

Over the past 10–20 years there has been a massive increase in type 2 diabetes in both the developed and undeveloped world (the 'diabetes epidemic'). This is forecast to increase even more rapidly in the next 10–20 years, by around 25% in Europe but about 50% in Asia. The disease, formerly rare in the young, is occurring more frequently in adolescents and young adults, especially when they are overweight and inactive.

### 1.25  How and why is the prevalence of diabetes changing?

The number of people with diabetes is increasing in most developed and developing countries by about 3–8% per year. For example, in the Poole (UK) Diabetes Study between 1984 and 1996, there was a 7% annual increase in type 2 diabetes.[22] The greatest increase in prevalence is occurring in Asia, but all areas of the world are affected.

One detailed statistical projection over the next 10 years in New Zealand gives the reasons for the increase as:

- population size (30%)
- obesity (30%)
- ageing of the population (20%)
- changing ethnic mixes (11%)
- improved survival of people with diagnosed diabetes (9%).

The only really modifiable factor in this equation is obesity.

Major contributory factors in developing countries are the rapid changes in diet and physical activity that lead to significant obesity. Increasing wealth, improved food supplies and less reliance on hard physical labour to earn a living are important factors in the equation.

### 1.26  Is the prevalence of type 1 diabetes changing?

While less than the spectacular 'epidemic' of type 2 diabetes, over the last 20 years there has been a steady 2–3% annual rise in the incidence and prevalence of type 1 diabetes in most populations studied from South Island, New Zealand to the UK and Scandinavia. In some studies, the age at diagnosis is also getting younger, the incidence in under 5-year-olds increasing faster than in older age groups. There is no clear explanation for this phenomenon.

Worldwide there are significant differences in the incidence and prevalence of type 1 diabetes, being highest in European-originating populations at high latitudes (*Fig. 1.6*).

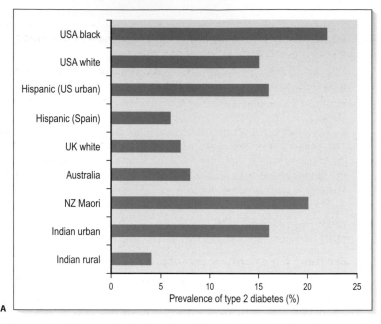

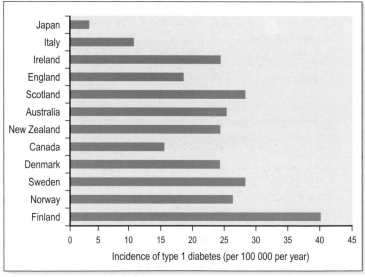

**Fig. 1.6A,** The prevalence of type 2 diabetes in different countries and groups. Data from multiple sources and estimated to 2004 levels. Note the urban:rural divide and the high levels in most of the ethnic groups described. **B,** The incidence of type 1 diabetes in some different countries. Data from multiple sources and estimated to 2004 levels.

### 1.27  What is likely to change in the next few years in diagnosis, screening and prevention of diabetes?

Diagnostic criteria for diabetes, IGT and IFG will probably be further revised. HbA1c may become acceptable as a component of the criteria, possibly with a different cut-off level than the upper end of the reference range.

The metabolic syndrome will become increasingly important and there may well be a 'metabolic index' which reflects macrovascular risk, whereas the HbA1c reflects microvascular risk. Population screening for diabetes may become validated as part of an overall risk assessment profile for all micro- and macrovascular disease.

Hopefully, we will see the development of effective and affordable population strategies to prevent type 2 diabetes, and a major breakthrough in prevention of type 1 diabetes.

### 1.28  Are there any important recent journal articles?

Yes, some particular reports of note, among thousands published, are:

- The causes and prevention of type 1 diabetes have been well reviewed,[27] together with the result of the European Nicotinamide Diabetes Intervention Trial (ENDIT) showing no benefit to nicotinamide [28]
- New evidence on the possible cause of type 2 diabetes as being with mitochondria.[29,30]
- A number of articles on renal disease from pathology,[31] through new treatments[32] to end-stage renal failure.[33]

 **PATIENT QUESTIONS**

#### 1.29   How can you be certain I have diabetes?

The diagnostic levels for diagnosing diabetes have been carefully set by the World Health Organization (WHO). These experts based their decisions on many detailed research studies. These had shown that, over the years, diabetes causes damage to areas of the body, particularly the eyes, kidneys and nerves but also the blood supply to the heart, brain and legs – these are known as the long-term complications of diabetes (*see also* Qs 2.14–2.17). The studies looked at a large number of people who had their blood sugar (glucose) levels measured at the start of the study and were then examined regularly to see if they had developed any of the long-term complications of diabetes. These showed that only when the blood sugar level was above a certain level did people develop some of these complications of diabetes.

PATIENT QUESTIONS

The WHO expert team therefore used these levels to decide the 'cut-off' point for diabetes. If your doctor has found that your blood sugar is in the range for diabetes, you will be at risk of developing these long-term complications irrespective of whether you feel unwell or not. As there are effective ways to prevent or delay these problems if treated early, it is most important that you receive care and treatment to lower your blood sugar and to detect any early damage before it becomes permanent.

### 1.30   Why have I got type 2 diabetes?

It is not always possible to explain why an individual patient develops type 2 diabetes. Factors that may be relevant include obesity, family history, and other diseases already present.

Being overweight makes a person more resistant to their own insulin, and the pancreas has to work harder to produce enough insulin to keep blood sugar levels in the normal range. In some susceptible people, especially those with a family history of diabetes, the strain of the extra work on the pancreas leads to exhaustion of the organ with time: too little insulin is then made and diabetes develops.

### 1.31   Will I need insulin?

In type 1 diabetes the answer is yes. Most patients have a considerable fear of injecting but, once they have got over the hurdle of starting, find it much easier with modern pens and needles than they expected.

For type 2 diabetes, the honest answer is also, yes – probably – in the long term. Insulin secretion gradually decreases with time, and diet and lifestyle, and then tablets, become less effective. The time between diagnosis and insulin being needed varies widely between different people. A recent UK study found that, 5 years after diagnosis of type 2 diabetes, one in six people was being treated with insulin.

# Natural history, glycaemic control and complications

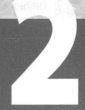

## NATURAL HISTORY OF GLYCAEMIC CONTROL

### 2.1    What is the natural history of type 2 diabetes?

Only in the past 10 years has this become really clear. Type 2 diabetes is a progressive disorder with insulin secretion declining over the years, whereas insulin resistance changes relatively little, unless there are major changes in lifestyle and/or body weight. This is best illustrated by the UKPDS.[1] After the initial response to lifestyle and dietary changes, followed by the introduction of hypoglycaemic therapy, there is a relentless drift upward in HbA1c despite the continuation of these therapies (*Fig. 2.1*). Obviously hypoglycaemic therapy will need to be increased if good glycaemic control is to be maintained. Indeed, most patients will require insulin replacement therapy in due course if they survive long enough.

The rate of decline in pancreatic beta-cell function is variable, but tends to be consistent within an individual. In general, younger patients show a

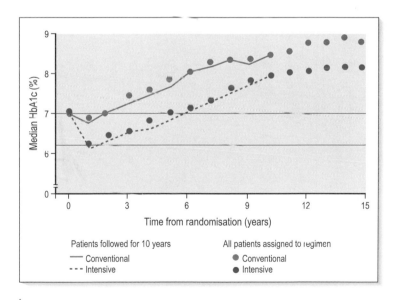

**Fig. 2.1**  The change of HbA1c over time in the intensive and conventional groups in the UKPDS. While there is a 0.9% separation between the groups there is an inexorable worsening of glycaemic control in both over time despite the target of fasting blood glucose below 6 mmol/l. (From UK Prospective Diabetes Study Group[1] with permission from Elsevier.)

more rapid deterioration, as do those who are of normal or low body weight. Leaner patients have less insulin resistance (their initial insulin secretion is presumably more impaired) and most studies have shown that they progress more rapidly to requiring insulin than those obese patients who have relatively well-preserved insulin secretion but marked insulin resistance. However, in the 5-year follow-up of the Poole (UK) cohort, the proportion of patients progressing to insulin was actually highest (13%) in those with BMI >35 kg/m² compared to 8% in those with BMI < 35 kg/m². Insulin resistance may be a powerful 'exhauster' of beta-cell function.

The mean time from diagnosis to institution of insulin treatment is about 7–10 years though diabetes has often been present for 5–10 years before diagnosis, implying 12–20 years of disease progression before insulin is currently instituted. With recent reductions in target values for glycaemic control, this time is likely to shorten.

It is important to recognize that any of the complications can be present at the time of diagnosis. This is commonest with eye disease (*Fig. 2.2*) but patients can and do present with foot ulcers and infections and, occasionally, with diabetic renal disease (*see Q. 2.14*).

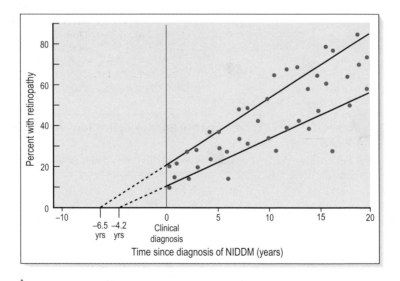

**Fig. 2.2** The prevalence of retinopathy with time after diagnosis in two studies of cohorts of type 2 diabetes. The implication is that retinopathy has been present for 4–6 years before diagnosis and, by implication, diabetes has been present for several more years than that. NIDDM, non-insulin dependent diabetes mellitus. (Copyright © 2003 American Diabetes Association. From Diabetes Care, Vol. 26, 2003; 1731–1737. Reprinted with permission from the American Diabetes Association.)

## 2.2     What about type 1 diabetes?

Only about 10% of islet-cell function remains when patients become symptomatic (*see* Q. *1.19*), and this usually disappears over the following few years. Often there is a period, a few weeks to several months after starting on insulin, when insulin requirements may fall – the 'honeymoon period' – which probably relates to partial beta-cell recovery when glucose control has been restored. Though usually short, it sometimes lasts a few years in older patients, but always ends with increasing insulin requirements – the average insulin dose in type 1 diabetes is eventually about 0.7 units/kg/day.

## THE EVIDENCE BEHIND GOOD GLYCAEMIC CONTROL

## 2.3     How strong is the evidence that good glycaemic control reduces microvascular and macrovascular outcomes in type 2 diabetes?

Over the past 10 years the evidence has become overwhelming. Three major studies – one in type 1 diabetes (DCCT[2]) and two in type 2 diabetes (Kumamoto[3] and UKPDS[1,4]) – have proved the case for microvascular complications. The epidemiological data in UKPDS, but not the randomised groups, showed a link between macrovascular events and level of glycaemic control. These three landmark studies have confirmed a wealth of other evidence that glycaemic control is the largest single factor affecting microvascular outcomes in diabetes. *Table 2.1* shows the major features of the three studies.

## 2.4     What did the Diabetes Control and Complications Trial (DCCT) show?

This massive study of younger patients with type 1 diabetes, diagnosed for between 1 and 15 years, was carried out between 1986 and 1992.[2] Patients were randomised to either intensive control (multiple insulin injections or pump therapy) or to conventional treatment (not more than two injections daily). Intensive control involved intervention by educators, dietitians, psychologists and doctors with frequent telephone contact and visits. HbA1c was reduced by 2%. Both the development of all new microvascular complications and the progression of early retinopathy were reduced by 40–70%, all of which were highly significant both statistically and clinically. The study was not powered to look at macrovascular outcomes, though there was a trend in this direction.

## 2.5     What was the Kumamoto study?

This Japanese study included middle-aged patients with type 2 diabetes of normal weight rather than obese.[3] Randomisation was to intensive or

**TABLE 2.1 Table of the major features of the three main control and complication studies**

|  | DCCT | Kumamoto | UKPDS |
|---|---|---|---|
| Report date | 1993 | 1995 | 1998 |
| Country | North America | Japan | Britain |
| Patients | Type 1, young | Type 2 | Type 2 |
| Groups | Uncomplicated or early complications | Uncomplicated Early complications | Newly diagnosed |
| Interventions | Intensive vs conventional | Intensive vs conventional insulin | Intensive vs conventional, but multiple groups |
| Study duration | Up to 6.5 years | 6 years | Up to 15 years |
| Number of patients | 1441 type 1 | 110 non-obese type 2 | 5200 type 2, mainly overweight |
| Insulin dose | 0.7 units/kg | 0.4 units/kg | – |
| Outcomes | Microvascular | Microvascular | Microvascular and macrovascular |
| HbA1c in two groups | 7% vs 9% | 7% vs 9% | 7% vs 7.9% |
| Nephropathy | Reduced | Reduced | Reduced |
| Retinopathy | Reduced | Reduced | Reduced |
| Neuropathy | Reduced | Reduced | Reduced |
| Macrovascular events | Not significant (not powered); weak trend towards reduction | Not significant (not powered); weak trend towards reduction | Borderline significance except for metformin in obese; epidemiological analysis showed relationship |

conventional insulin therapy, and microvascular and macrovascular outcomes were measured in a very similar way to DCCT. The HbA1c differences were almost identical to the DCCT, falling from around 9 to 7% in the intensive group, maintained for the course of the study. Once again microvascular outcomes were improved, as detailed in *Table 2.1*; the study was not powered to measure macrovascular outcomes, though there was a trend in this direction.[3]

## 2.6 Why was the United Kingdom Prospective Diabetes Study (UKPDS) so important?

This landmark 10-year study (*Box 2.1*) involved 5000 patients, recruited from newly diagnosed type 2 diabetic patients in 23 centres in the UK. As

---

**BOX 2.1  Major outcomes of the UKPDS**

*Glycaemic control*[1,4]
- ■ Intensive control reduced overall microvascular complications, especially retinopathy
- ■ Intensive control did not significantly reduce macrovascular outcomes or mortality; risk of myocardial infarction was of borderline significance
- ■ Intensive control with metformin in the obese subgroup reduced overall and diabetes-related mortality; this was not so for sulphonylureas and insulin
- ■ Weight was increased in all but the metformin group, but quality of life was not altered

*Blood pressure*[5]
- ■ Tight BP control reduced diabetes-related mortality
- ■ Tight BP control reduced overall complications
- ■ Both captopril and atenolol were equally effective
- ■ BP lowering by 13/5 mmHg achieved a greater fall in complications than the 0.9% reduction in HbA1c

*Epidemiological analysis*[6,7]
- ■ Later analysis by achieved not allocated levels of HbA1c and BP showed clear continuous relationships
- ■ No lower threshold was seen for either glycaemic or BP relationships

---

the protocol was designed in the late 1970s, the intensive therapy group (which used chlorpropromide, glibenclamide, insulin, or metformin for the obese) was not optimised by modern standards and a comparatively small HbA1c difference of 0.9% ensued. There was a major effect seen on the microvascular outcomes, but macrovascular outcomes were not significantly different.

Macrovascular outcomes were, however, clearly reduced in the subgroup of obese patients treated with metformin,[4] where there were major reductions in myocardial infarction and mortality (*Fig. 2.3*).

In both the Kumamoto and UKPDS studies, hypoglycaemia was commoner in the intensively treated groups, but at a much lower rate in both groups than the three-fold excess in type 1 diabetes in the DCCT.

In addition to these three pivotal studies, there are numerous smaller studies, nearly all showing similar trends or outcomes, and a meta-analysis[8] clearly confirms this for microvascular disease (*Fig. 2.4*).

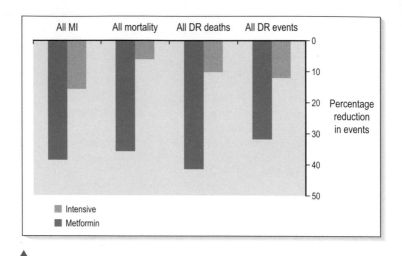

▲

**Fig. 2.3** A comparison of the benefits from metformin in the obese group in UKPDS and other intensive treatments (sulphonylureas and insulin), compared with the conventional group (baseline). DR, diabetes related; MI, myocardial infarction.

## 2.7 What are the risks associated with improved glycaemic control?

The major concern is hypoglycaemia, especially if severe (defined as needing the assistance of a third party to remedy, *see Ch. 7*). This is the major limitation of intensive treatment in diabetes, and increases exponentially as mean HbA1c falls (*see Q. 7.12 and Fig. 7.2*). The frequency of hypoglycaemia at any given HbA1c is much greater in type 1 than in type 2 diabetes. Hypoglycaemia does not occur when metformin or thiazolidinediones (TZDs, 'glitazones') are used alone (*see Q. 7.6*). There is evidence that hypoglycaemia is reduced with more modern insulin regimens, especially with ultra-short-acting insulins (e.g. NovoRapid/Humalog). Recent general improvements in glycaemic control have increased awareness of hypoglycaemia and its avoidance. Better understanding of the mechanisms and improved education about self-management have meant that serious hypoglycaemia is much reduced from DCCT days but still represents a significant limitation.

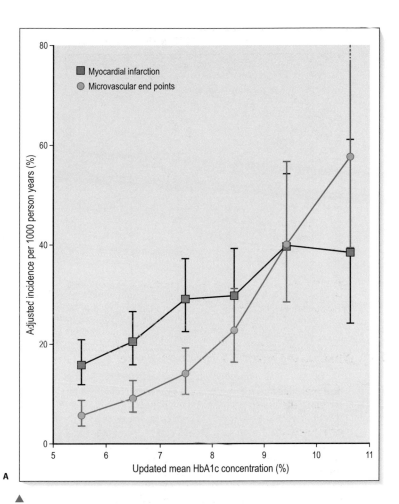

**A**

**Fig. 2.4 A**, The relationship between mean glycaemic control in UKPDS and incidence rates of microvascular disease and myocardial infarction. **B**, The relationship between achieved blood pressure and rate of myocardial infarction in UKPDS (microvascular outcomes included for comparison). (**A**, from Stratton et al.[7]; **B**, from Adler et al.[6], both with permission from the BMJ Publishing Group.)

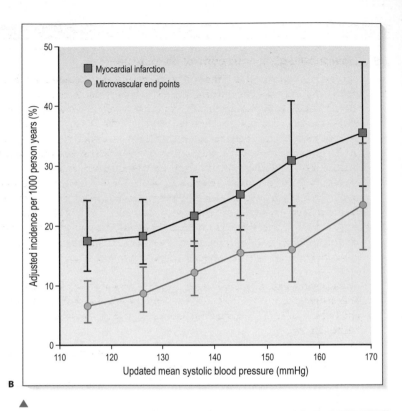

**B**

**Fig. 2.4 (Cont'd). B**, The relationship between achieved blood pressure and rate of myocardial infarction in UKPDS (microvascular outcomes included for comparison). (**A**, from Stratton et al.[7]; **B**, from Adler et al.[6], both with permission from the BMJ Publishing Group.)

Rapid improvement in glycaemic control may worsen retinopathy in some patients with type 1 or type 2 diabetes over a period of 1–2 years, though the longer-term outcome of improved control becomes clearly beneficial after around 3 years. This usually occurs in patients where control has been consistently poor (HbA1c >10%) and is dramatically improved within months. There is anecdotal evidence that acute painful neuropathy may similarly worsen if glycaemic control is suddenly and rapidly improved, but there is no clear evidence that a similar situation occurs in renal disease.

## MEASURING CONTROL AND SETTING TARGETS

### 2.8 How should glycaemic control be measured?

For the long term, HbA1c is the best currently available method though it is not infallible and has some variation that is *not* purely due to changes in mean blood glucose (BG) levels. Most guidelines recommend 3–6-monthly checks for patients with type 1 diabetes, and 6-monthly for those with type 2, possibly more often in patients on insulin. That said, clinical conditions such as change in circumstances or therapy may sensibly determine more frequent measurements, while long-term stability might allow longer intervals.

On a day-to-day basis, many patients with diabetes perform self-testing of BG levels, especially when on insulin, and this is used for adjustment of their treatment. The evidence supporting the value of self blood-testing alone is weak, as most studies have been in the context of overall intensive treatment rather than BG monitoring alone. There is little evidence on the efficacy of self-testing from which to make firm recommendations (*see Q. 11.2*).

Most guidelines empirically recommend testing of BG on some days both before meals and 1.5–2 hours after meals to establish both the lower and higher limits. These suggestions are based on expert consensus, not hard evidence:

- ■ For patients on diet alone, metformin or thiazolidinediones, it is usually sufficient to record a fasting and post-prandial BG or undertake urine testing on 2–3 days a week while stable. Even less frequent testing may be appropriate.
- ■ For those on sulphonylureas or meglitinides, occasional samples should be taken at times of hypoglycaemia risk (e.g. pre-lunch, pre-dinner, pre-bedtime and/or during the night).
- ■ For those on nocturnal insulin, some fasting samples are essential and some later daytime ones will often show the periods of worst control.
- ■ Twice daily and more complex insulin regimens need pre- or post-meal samples, up to two to four per day, though not every day.
- ■ In pregnancy, and those at high risk of hypoglycaemia or treated with multiple insulin injections and food adjustment, four to seven readings daily are often needed.

### 2.9 What actually is HbA1c?

HbA1c, glycated haemoglobin (formerly called glycosylated haemoglobin), is the most widely used measure of long-term glycaemic control. It is formed by the passive glycation of the haemoglobin molecule, which is dependent on the prevailing BG concentration, with the reaction being partly irreversible. It correlates well with average BG concentrations, which in the normal situation will relate most accurately to fasting BG rather than post-prandial levels. HbA1c reflects BG levels over approximately 2 months. It is the outcome measure used in all the major studies described above, where it showed a high rate of correlation with microvascular outcomes.

### 2.10 Is HbA1c really an adequate measure of overall glycaemic control? How does it relate to pre- and post-prandial glucose levels?

HbA1c does have problem areas. First, there are small but significant genetic and familial variations, which make it less precise than ideal. Second, there are a number of different analytical methods that do not give identical results. All local laboratories should give clear reference ranges; laboratories are increasingly reporting 'DCCT-aligned' results, which should give values of 4.5–6.1%. Finally, certain haemoglobinopathies and conditions affecting red-cell survival will alter the result with some methods. This includes people with anaemia and chronic renal failure. HbA1c is not useful in patients after a recent blood transfusion.

Additionally there are problems with standardisation of any HbA1c assay, and new conventions may soon be introduced which may result in changes to the reference range. At present for most purposes, results need to be expressed in terms of a DCCT-aligned method.

### 2.11 How do HbA1c levels equate to mean plasma glucose?

*Figure 2.5* gives a rough guide for HbA1c assays calibrated to the DCCT standard.

### 2.12 What glycaemic target should I be aiming for in my patients with diabetes?

In the DCCT, Kumamoto and UKPDS studies, the mean HbA1c in the intensively treated patients was in the range 7.0–7.2%. The groups did encompass patients with readings as low as 5.5 and above 8.5%. Epidemiological analysis from UKPDS, but not a controlled trial, suggests benefit was greatest when the HbA1c was lowest. There is little evidence to suggest a specific threshold below which complications do not occur, though there is a positive exponential relationship between increasing HbA1c and the absolute risk of complications. The reduction in absolute risk is therefore greater for a reduction in HbA1c from 10 to 8% than for 8 to 6%. There is some suggestion that macrovascular risk may continue to fall rather further to lower levels of HbA1c.

Different authoritative guidelines suggest a variety of HbA1c targets including <6.5%, <7% and an individualised level between 6.5 and 7.5%.[9–12] All are agreed that lower is better, as long as hypoglycaemia is not a major problem. This makes a lower target potentially more achievable for patients

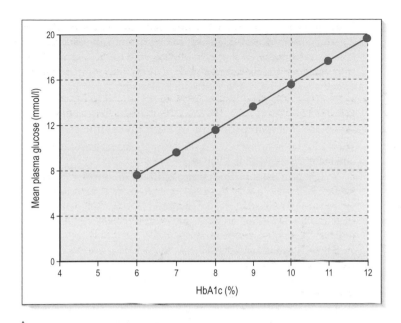

**Fig. 2.5** The correlation between HbA1c (DCCT-aligned method) and mean blood glucose. This is, of course, a mean and associated with a range at any value.

managed with lifestyle measures or on metformin or glitazones as hypoglycaemia is not a consequence of intensive treatment, compared to patients on insulin or a sulphonylurea/meglitinide where hypoglycaemia can be significant. Other factors that should be taken into account include age, overall microvascular and macrovascular risk, the presence of complications of diabetes or other co-morbidities and, of course, patient choice and psychosocial circumstances such as living alone and frailty.[13] The authors' departments use the HbA1c targets outlined in *Table 2.2* as a guide.

### TABLE 2.2  Suggested HbA1c targets

| Patient group | Approximate target | Action if |
| --- | --- | --- |
| Diet alone, metformin or TZD alone | <6.5% | > 6.8–7% |
| Sulphonylurea/meglitinide | <7% | > 7.5% |
| Insulin alone or in combination | <7.5% | > approximately 8% |

Finally, there needs to be a recognition that current treatment of diabetes is far from perfect and achieving excellent glycaemic control may not always be possible.[13] This certainly seems to be the case with patients with significant insulin resistance where increasing insulin doses result in little change in HbA1c. The 'best achievable' control may be the target as any reduction in HbA1c will be valuable, especially from very high levels.

### 2.13 What are the main problems of tight glycaemic control?

The frequency of hypoglycaemia has been discussed above, and further questions are answered in Chapter 7.[14,15]

Weight gain is a common adverse outcome of intensive insulin treatment in both types of diabetes. Apart from diet or metformin treatment alone, all other treatment options for type 2 diabetes lead to weight gain – tightening up glycaemic control seems to exacerbate this problem, particularly when insulin is added.

For every individual with diabetes, the potential benefits of intensive glycaemic control should be balanced against the actual or expected risks. Many patients have conditions which limit the degree of improvement in glycaemic control. These include particularly those patients with hypoglycaemic unawareness (*see Q. 7.5*), those who have frequent or severe hypoglycaemia (especially where driving or occupational safety is an issue) and those who live alone, or might suffer severe injury if there was major hypoglycaemia.

The rigorous lifestyle, and the need for frequent monitoring and treatment adjustment may not be on the patient's personal agenda. Insufficient attention has been given to patient choice in deciding what risk of complications and hypoglycaemia they wish to accept. Not surprisingly, significant hypoglycaemia causes a reduction in quality of life, whereas there appear to be improvements in overall quality of life with better glycaemic control if hypoglycaemia is avoided.

## COMPLICATIONS

### 2.14 How likely are the different complications of diabetes?

This depends upon the duration of diabetes (including the period of unrecognized hyperglycaemia in type 2 diabetes) and multiple other factors, including mean glycaemic control, BP and smoking habits. Hypertension, particularly uncontrolled, is significantly related to an increased risk of micro- and macrovascular complications (*see Fig. 2.4B*). Some basic facts are as follows:

■ *Eye disease*: After 20–25 years, some mild diabetic changes will occur in most patients. More serious changes needing laser treatment are seen in about 20–25%.

- *Renal disease*: Early renal changes (microalbuminuria) are seen in 25% of patients after 10 years, with more severe signs such as proteinuria and kidney failure occurring in 5% and < 1%, respectively. Renal disease appears commoner in some non-European groups.
- *Nervous damage*: Most people will have some minor changes, often with no symptoms, after 20–25 years; severe damage leading to gangrene or amputation occurs in less than 5%.
- *Heart attack and stroke*: These are the major killers in Western society, even more so in type 2 diabetes than in the non-diabetic population.

Obviously outcomes for recently diagnosed patients will not be available for many years but there are emerging data suggesting that many complications are being delayed, if not totally prevented – this probably relates to improved treatment of both BG and other risk factors.[16–21]

## 2.15  Do microvascular and macrovascular risks move in parallel?

In all studies where these can be compared (especially UKPDS), there is the same overall relationship: that of better glycaemic control being associated with fewer microvascular and macrovascular outcomes, but with increased hypoglycaemic episodes. However, in type 2 diabetes there is a relatively high incidence of macrovascular events in even the best-controlled patients, presumably reflecting that these events (e.g. myocardial infarction and stroke) also occur in those with normoglycaemia, while diabetic microvascular complications are limited to those with diabetes! In many ways, this is similar to the relationship of macrovascular disease with impaired glucose tolerance (IGT), impaired fasting glucose (IFG) and the metabolic syndrome. It lends further support to the suggestion that macrovascular outcomes might show continuing benefit from lowering BG into the normal range if this can be safely achieved, while microvascular complications are virtually absent at these levels.

## 2.16  Is there any symptomatic or simple clinical way to detect the onset of complications?

To a large extent, no. Apart from occasional cases of painful neuropathy, most of the important complications cause no significant symptoms in their early or even advanced stages, and can only be detected by deliberate screening, as illustrated in *Table 2.3*.

## 2.17  Are any of the complications of diabetes reversible?

Both yes and no is the answer here. At the severe end of the spectrum, renal impairment, visual loss and severe neuropathy rarely regress significantly as anatomical damage has already occurred – prevention of further deterioration is usually the best that can be achieved. Exceptions are the acute neuropathies (e.g. some painful neuropathies, cranial or

**TABLE 2.3 Diabetic complications, symptomatology and detection**

| Complication | Symptomatology | Detection |
|---|---|---|
| Retinopathy | Visual acuity often maintained until late stages | Photography Ophthalmoscopy |
| Nephropathy | No symptoms until late-stage renal failure | Microalbuminuria Serum creatinine |
| Neuropathy | Rare painful neuropathy, some vaguely symptomatic, often asymptomatic | Filament sensation Biothesiometry |

mononeuropathies) which are usually time-limited with substantial or total recovery. Occasionally short-term deterioration in renal and retinal function is reversed.

At an earlier stage, the news is better. Retinal exudates and haemorrhages come and go, and can be reduced by good glycaemic and anti-hypertensive treatment or, later, by laser therapy. Microalbuminuria can improve with better control and angiotensin converting enzyme (ACE) inhibition, especially if it has been present only a short time.

## PROGNOSIS

### 2.18 What is the prognosis for type 2 diabetes?

'No-one knows' is the only honest answer we can currently give for recently diagnosed patients – only with the passage of time will we know for certain. There are few up-to-date reliable data. If you compare a 'typical' overweight middle-aged patient with type 2 diabetes around 1980–1985 and in 2003, the contrasts in treatment are evident (*Table 2.4*).

**TABLE 2.4 Contrast in treatment of diabetes between 1980–1985 and 2003**

| Treatment | 1980s | 2000s |
|---|---|---|
| Glycaemic control | Sulphonylureas first Late insulin: ? when HbA1c >10% | Metformin first Early insulin: ? when HbA1c >8.5% |
| Blood pressure | If above ~160/100 mmHg | If cardiovascular risk high |
| Lipid lowering | Only if cholesterol over 8 | Probably statin or fibrate |
| Anti-platelet | No | Aspirin if high risk |
| Renal protection/ high risk | No | Angiotensin converting enzyme inhibitor |

Unfavourable signs for prognosis, apart from poor glycaemic control, are development of microalbuminuria, proteinuria or renal dysfunction; continued smoking and poor adherence to therapy.

## 2.19 What is the prognosis for type 1 diabetes?

There is no doubt that type 1 diabetes substantially shortens life expectancy, by up to 15 years in some studies,[22] but again there is promising evidence that the situation is improving (*Fig. 2.6*).

It will of course be decades before we can be really sure whether this involves permanent prevention or just delays in complications and mortality, but even delay is well worthwhile. Causes of death in type 1 diabetes in younger patients (below age 35) are primarily metabolic – ketoacidosis and hypoglycaemia – after which cardiovascular and renal causes increasingly predominate. With renal replacement therapy many, if not most, of the deaths are also cardiovascular. The major determinant of

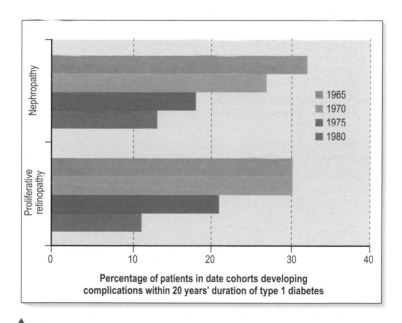

**Fig. 2.6** The prevalence of nephropathy and proliferative retinopathy in type 1 diabetes in successive 5-year cohorts. Both complications show progressive falls in prevalence over 20 years.

premature death is the development of any renal damage, mortality increasing progressively along the scale:

normoalbuminuria → microalbuminuria → proteinuria → raised creatinine → end-stage renal failure.

Perhaps most worrying is the excess of deaths seen in women even before the menopause, when non-diabetic women appear protected against coronary and cerebrovascular disease. This protection is lost in women with diabetes and they have a very high relative risk of death, though the absolute level is still not high if they do not have any renal involvement.

 **PATIENT QUESTIONS**

### 2.20 Can I not feel when my sugar is high or low?

The answer here is both yes and no. Most people with diabetes recognize symptoms of *low* blood sugar (usually 4 mmol/l and under), and are able to treat the episode quickly. At the *high* end, symptoms (often thirst and tiredness) are not recognized unless blood glucose levels are over 12–15 mmol/l, higher than the levels one would want to see. Several studies have shown that most people cannot accurately estimate their own blood glucose within the range of 4–15 mmol/l, though there may be some rare individuals who can.

Low blood glucose levels (below 4 mmol/l) are commoner in patients on insulin than those on sulphonylureas (e.g. glibenclamide, gliclazide, glipizide), meglitinides (repaglinide or nateglinide) and rarely occur in those on metformin alone. Individuals tend to have their own pattern of specific warning symptoms of hypoglycaemia, but even then recognition of hypoglycaemia can be delayed if 'hypos' occur too often. The body seems to become used to lower glucose levels. The warning symptoms do not occur until the blood glucose level is much lower (around 2 mmol/l). It is important to confirm blood glucose readings at the time of some hypoglycaemic episodes (if you have any), and essential if you are driving, operating machinery or alone in a position of responsibility (e.g. caring for children).

Similarly it is worth checking your blood glucose about 2 hours after a main meal, even if you don't have symptoms. Some people will be surprised how high the blood glucose can go without any obvious symptoms.

### 2.21 What does HbA1c mean?

HbA1c is shorthand for a special sort of haemoglobin (the red blood pigment) that has glucose stuck to it. The more glucose there is in the blood, the more 'sticks' to the haemoglobin. This special 'glycated' haemoglobin can then be measured as a proportion of the total haemoglobin, and this level reflects the average glucose over the past 6–8 weeks. For a rough 'translation' see *Figure 2.5*.

### 2.22 Why does my doctor want my glucose levels even lower?

The lower your average blood glucose (the HbA1c, which measures this over the previous 6–8 weeks), the lower is your risk of eye, kidney and nerve complications and also of heart attack and stroke. Obviously your medical team wants this as low as possible – most guidelines now recommend an HbA1c of 7% or less. For patients whose diabetes is controlled on diet alone or on metformin this is a good target as there is no risk of hypoglycaemia.

### 2.23 What if I can't achieve better control?

Don't give up. Not everyone can, and this has to be faced and worked on with your care team. However, any small improvement is well worthwhile, even from an HbA1c of 11 to 10%, or 10 to 9%.

Additionally there are ways to detect any early damage and these checks for eyes, kidneys and nerves may need to be more frequent if control cannot be improved. Treatment of early signs of damage and any risk factors such as high BP or blood fats (cholesterol) can also prevent serious complications developing.

# Clinical presentation and initial management of diabetes

# 3

## PROBLEMS AFTER DIAGNOSIS

## OTHER ASPECTS OF LIFESTYLE

## SYMPTOMS OF DIABETES

### 3.1 What causes the symptoms of thirst, polyuria, tiredness and weight loss in diabetes?

Hyperglycaemia and failure to convert glucose into energy  are the root cause of the symptoms. The glycosuria and accompanying salt loss may lead to mild dehydration and compensatory thirst and, with heavy glycosuria, a significant amount of energy is lost in the urine hence the weight loss. Utilising energy depends on insulin promoting glucose uptake into cells which, with absolute or relative insulin insufficiency, leads to suboptimal functioning of cells, particularly in muscle. Not surprisingly, the patient feels a sense of fatigue and general lethargy. These typical symptoms occur not only at the time of diagnosis, but also during periods of poor glycaemic control.

### 3.2 Why do some people have no symptoms at the time of diagnosis?

Patients' sensitivities clearly vary and symptoms of diabetes may be non-specific. Feelings of tiredness, lethargy and irritability are not uncommon but patients often blame other causes such as depression, poor sleep or increasing age – 'I just thought I was getting older'.

Minor derangement of plasma glucose (PG) produces few symptoms – there is no exact 'cut-off' but levels persistently above 12–15 mmol/l are usually associated with clear symptoms, and even lower levels may give rise to mild symptoms or tiredness.

Development of type 2 diabetes is usually very slow with the transition from normal glucose levels to hyperglycaemia over many months or years. Thus patients fail to detect the subtle change from health to illness. It is not uncommon for people to deny any symptoms at diagnosis. But, after establishing good glycaemic control, they frequently report feeling much better, realising that they had failed to recognise the effects of diabetes previously.

In the future, as further screening for diabetes occurs, more cases will be detected at an earlier stage when symptoms are less severe. In some areas, over 50% of cases are currently detected by routine testing or screening of high-risk individuals.

### 3.3 My patient presented a week after a minor road traffic accident with type 2 diabetes and is convinced that the accident caused her diabetes. Is this possible?

This is a common assumption among patients when some life event precedes the diagnosis of diabetes. However, it is most unlikely to be the actual cause, unless there was pancreatic injury which is rare and clinically obvious. The natural history of type 2 diabetes is for a long period of progression from normal glucose levels to hyperglycaemia as pancreatic function gradually deteriorates. The stress of a road traffic accident or other life event might lead to a sudden increase in plasma glucose as circulating adrenaline and catecholamines antagonise the action of insulin and demands on a failing pancreas are rapidly increased. The sudden rise in PG levels can produce the typical symptoms of diabetes and alert the patient to the problem.

Without the life event, the patient would have developed diabetes at some stage over the next few months or years; the accident has merely precipitated the diagnosis. The chance of being diagnosed is increased as the patient is more likely to see a health professional and/or have investigations after an accident. Often in this situation there is evidence such as old records, which show marginally abnormal PG levels beforehand, or the presence of complications indicating previously undiagnosed diabetes.

In type 1 diabetes, where the time to diagnosis of diabetes is much shorter, it is still unlikely that a life event actually caused diabetes. In longitudinal family studies, islet cell and other antibodies (the hallmark of the autoimmune process associated with the development of type 1 diabetes) are detectable in some patients for years before the diagnosis. The process leading to the development of diabetes thus started long before the event, though there is some study evidence that life events precede/precipitate the diagnosis but not the disease process.

## INVESTIGATIONS OF THE CAUSE OF DIABETES

### 3.4　What investigations are required to look for a cause?

For most patients, no specific investigations are required. There are a number of causes of secondary diabetes (*see Box 1.1*). Taking a careful history of previous illness and family history of diabetes will help to identify patients with cystic fibrosis, pancreatitis, pancreatic surgery and possible genetic causes. A high index of suspicion needs to be maintained for rare endocrine causes such as Cushing's disease and acromegaly. Haemochromatosis characteristically causes skin pigmentation but may be difficult to spot; abnormal liver function tests may be a possible indicator.

### 3.5　In which patients are further investigations worthwhile?

Investigations may be appropriate if it is not clear whether patients have type 1 or type 2 diabetes. Islet-cell antibodies are present in up to 90% of young people with type 1 diabetes, though glutamic acid dehydrogenase antibodies are more useful in older patients with possible type 1 diabetes/latent autoimmune diabetes in adults (LADA). While they do not always indicate type 1 diabetes, they do predict an early transition to insulin treatment.

Detailed family histories are also valuable. In type 2 diabetes, a search for a genetic cause may be worthwhile where there is a family history and the patient is of European origin, aged <45 years, BMI <27 kg/m² with normal BP and triglyceride levels – in other words few characteristics of the 'metabolic syndrome'.

## 3.6  Can pancreatic cancer underlie a diagnosis of diabetes?

Rarely. Some people worry that diabetes may be the first presentation of pancreatic cancer. This is fortunately rare since this unpleasant cancer usually presents with abdominal symptoms (e.g. pain, jaundice, anorexia, weight loss) long before diabetes is produced. If any of these features is prominent, a full physical examination is vital, followed by an abdominal pancreatic and liver ultrasound scan.

However, patients with chronic pancreatitis who have an increased incidence of pancreatic cancer may already have significantly reduced pancreatic endocrine function. It is therefore possible – but unusual – for diabetes to present in this way.

## TYPE 2 AND TYPE 1 DIABETES

### 3.7  How do you distinguish between type 1 and type 2 diabetes in practice?

Normally, history, age and clinical features make this easy to distinguish (*Table 3.1*). However, type 1 diabetes can occur at any age and maintaining a strong index of suspicion is important. Consider the possibility in any patient with a short history and/or significant non-deliberate weight loss. Testing the urine for the presence of ketones, which would suggest insulin deficiency, is the next step. Ketones (especially trace amounts) are also seen during starvation so it is worth checking that the patient is eating normally.

Occasionally, the onset of type 1 diabetes is slow, especially in the older age group who may have had symptoms for many months or even years. These patients are not usually overweight but may have no urinary ketones and PG levels are not particularly high, perhaps only in the range 12–25 mmol/l. There is still some insulin secretion, which prevents ketosis developing. However, with time, insulin secretion deteriorates and such patients eventually and inevitably become truly insulin dependent. Sometimes, these patients can be treated initially with oral hypoglycaemic agents (OHAs). However, the transition to insulin treatment is often difficult psychologically for the patient. It is generally preferable to commence insulin (albeit in small doses) at diagnosis once type 1 diabetes has been confirmed.

**TABLE 3.1 Typical clinical features distinguishing type 1 and type 2 diabetes**

| Clinical feature | Type 1 diabetes | Type 2 diabetes |
|---|---|---|
| Commonest age | Mostly children to young adult<br>Can occur at any age | Middle age to elderly<br>5–10 years earlier in non-Europeans<br>Occasionally in teenagers/young adults, most often of Asian origin<br>Getting younger |
| History | Short, usually a few weeks/months | Long, usually many months to years |
| Presenting weight | Usually lean/normal<br>Losing weight recently | Usually overweight, often very obese |
| Symptoms | Intense thirst, polyuria, frequency, tiredness and recent weight loss | May be asymptomatic or have mild–moderate thirst, nocturia and tiredness |
| Signs | Sometimes dehydration | Rarely any specific |
| Urine | Heavy glycosuria<br>Often ketones | Glycosuria but no significant ketones |

### 3.8 If abnormal liver function tests are found at diagnosis of diabetes, what investigations should be done?

It is quite common to find mild to moderate abnormalities of LFTs, perhaps two to three times the upper range of normal, at diagnosis of diabetes, sometimes associated with hepatomegaly (*see also Qs 18.1 and 18.2*). The commonest cause is a fatty liver, now recognised in many people with the 'metabolic syndrome' (*see Q. 1.12*). More significant or persistent abnormalities of LFTs need further investigation, starting with a detailed history and including hepatic and biliary ultrasound to search for an underlying abnormality. Apart from fatty liver, common causes are:

- alcohol excess
- hepatitis B or C (common in Pacific Island and Maori populations)
- pancreatitis
- biliary disease
- haemochromatosis.

If there are clinical abnormalities – in particular physical signs of liver disease, abnormal clotting or low serum albumin – referral to a diabetologist or gastroenterologist is indicated. Serum ferritin may be misleading in the diagnosis of haemochromatosis as it is frequently raised at the time of diagnosis, being an acute-phase protein.

### 3.9 An initial lipid profile in a newly diagnosed patient showed a cholesterol level of 6.2 mmol/l and triglyceride level of 9.6 mmol/l. Should lipid-lowering treatment be started immediately?

Not unless there are pressing indications. Uncontrolled hyperglycaemia/insulin deficiency leads to derangement of lipids, particularly triglycerides. The first approach is dietary and then with OHAs if necessary. It is advisable to repeat the fasting lipid profile in 6–12 weeks, when reasonable control of PG levels has been achieved: the lipid abnormalities will often have dramatically improved, especially the triglycerides.

Occasionally extremely high triglyceride levels (>15 mmol/l) are seen and these patients can develop acute pancreatitis. Generally there is uncontrolled diabetes and often a high alcohol intake. Lipid levels should be brought down by strict diet and alcohol withdrawal – the profile should be repeated in 1–2 weeks, and an urgent referral made if it has not improved. If abdominal pain is prominent, referral should be immediate.

If the profile does not improve rapidly, the possibility of a genetic lipid disorder should be considered, so referral is appropriate.

## INITIAL MANAGEMENT ON DIAGNOSIS

### 3.10 What should I say and do at the first consultation to tell the patient they have diabetes?

Keep the consultation reasonably short and make the messages as simple but clear as possible:
- Give a brief explanation of diabetes based on high blood glucose levels, lack of insulin and resistance to its action.
- Reassure and emphasise the improvement in health that occurs once diabetes is well controlled.
- Initiate healthy dietary changes and give a simple diet information sheet if possible.
- Refer to a dietitian and/or educator.
- Do not discuss complications or long-term implications unless specifically asked.
- Outline what will happen over the next few weeks (*Box 3.1*) and arrange to see the patient again in a few days. Ask them to bring a partner or friend to the next consultation if they wish, and encourage them to write down a list of questions.
- If appropriate, give them details of a local or national diabetes association or a local support group (*see Appendix 3*).

BOX 3.1  **Steps in the initial management of type 2 diabetes: an example plan**

**Visit 1**
- Explain the diagnosis in simple terms
- Reassure and stress positive health benefits from controlling hyperglycaemia
- Start low sugar diet
- Arrange dietitian and educator appointments

**Visit 2**
- Take a full history including past illness, family history, smoking history, exercise and lifestyle
- Full examination including weight, height and calculate BMI, BP, feet and eyes (or arrange retinal screening)
- Check urine for proteinuria
- Arrange laboratory tests for HbA1c, fasting lipid profile, renal and liver function
- Explore anxieties and answer questions
- Reassure and explain management plan
- Commence home monitoring of diabetes
- Refer to specialist services if required and/or arrange follow-up in own practice

**Visit 3 (some weeks later)**
- Review symptoms and results of home monitoring
- Review results of previous laboratory investigations
- Start or adjust oral hypoglycaemic agents
- Listen to feelings and anxieties
- Arrange follow-up and next laboratory tests

## 3.11  What if this is type 1 diabetes?

Most aspects of management are the same, but with the obvious need to start insulin soon. Usually this will involve referral to specialist teams and should normally be an urgent phone call, with the patient being seen the same day. If this is not practicable and the specialist team agrees, the patient should be advised to:

- avoid all high glucose drinks and foods
- drink large amounts of water
- start blood glucose testing immediately if possible
- have immediate laboratory tests for glucose, electrolytes and creatinine, usually with a bicarbonate and serum ketones
- avoid exercise and stressful situations.

Young patients, those who are dehydrated or extremely hyperglycaemic (PG >30 mmol/l) should be seen immediately, as should anyone who lives alone or has poor family or social support. An immediate dose of subcutaneous insulin (e.g. 6–12 units) might be considered if full assessment and insulin treatment will be delayed.

Older patients may have type 1 diabetes, often called LADA (*see Q. 3.5*).

### 3.12 Which patients with newly diagnosed diabetes should be referred to specialist diabetes services and what are the timescales for doing so?

The organisation of diabetes services varies considerably in different areas and different countries, often with good reason as well as lack of resource! Some specialist diabetes services would expect referral of all newly diagnosed patients to undertake an initial assessment and to provide full education and treatment. In other areas, primary health care would undertake the initial assessment, education and management of many patients with type 2 diabetes, especially where the GP or practice nurse has experience in diabetes. All instances of newly diagnosed diabetes as outlined in *Box 3.2* should be referred for specialist assessment.

The UK does not define required timescales for waiting times for specialist diabetes services but other countries include such limits as:

■ *Same day*: newly diagnosed type 1 patients; type 2 patients with BG >25, ketonuria >1+ or intercurrent illness; acute visual loss; foot ulceration with infection.

■ *Within 1 week*: pregnancy (gestational or known diabetes); non-infected, non-acute foot ulceration; high-risk proliferative retinopathy.

---

### BOX 3.2 Cases of newly diagnosed diabetes to be referred for specialist assessment

■ All children and young people with newly diagnosed diabetes (urgent)

■ All patients with type 1 diabetes (usually urgent – *see Q. 3.11*)

■ All patients with type 2 diabetes with evidence of significant retinopathy, neuropathy or nephropathy *at the time of diagnosis*

■ All patients with type 2 diabetes with diabetic foot disease *at diagnosis*

■ All patients with newly diagnosed type 2 diabetes with significant other illness likely to cause problems with management (e.g. steroid treatment, chronic renal failure)

■ Any patient considering pregnancy within the next 12 months

■ *Within 4 weeks*: diabetic nephropathy (creatinine >200 µmol/l); painful neuropathy; newly diagnosed patients with existing complications; hypoglycaemia if severe or with unawareness.

■ *Within 12 weeks*: other instances of diabetic nephropathy; high-risk diabetic feet; hypoglycaemia; high cardiovascular risk patients; poor glycaemic control.

To conclude this section, examples of initial management on diagnosis are illustrated in *Case vignettes 3.1–3.3*.

### CASE VIGNETTE 3.1

A 55-year-old man presented with typical symptoms of diabetes. At diagnosis, his BMI is 34.2 kg/m² and the random laboratory PG is 29.2 mmol/l. Should an oral hypoglycaemic agent be started immediately?

*Comment*

The first question should be: 'What have you been drinking to ease your thirst and how much?'. These patients are often taking large quantities of 'Coke', other soft drinks and fruit juices labelled 'No added sugar' (the fruit fell off the tree loaded with sugar already!). Simply stopping these and changing to 'diet' drinks and water will often halve the PG level and improve symptoms within a few days. If you find he has not been taking a lot of sugary food or drinks in his diet, arrange to see him again in a few days. If there is no improvement in symptoms and PG remains high (>12–15 mmol/l) despite diet, then metformin should be commenced.

'Lite' drinks (e.g. Ribena Lite) are not recommended – they contain less sugar than Ribena but still a great deal; 'diet' drinks contain artificial sweetener that is appropriate in all normal amounts and contains no calories.

### CASE VIGNETTE 3.2

Two months ago a Pacific Island man aged 56 years presented with diabetes, obesity, a fasting PG of 16 mmol/l and HbA1c of 13.2%. He has made a lot of dietary and lifestyle changes with a weight loss of 6.5 kg. Metformin 500 mg twice daily was started after 1 month as he continued to be symptomatic and urine tests showed heavy glycosuria. He is now much better and urine tests are clear. Should his treatment now be increased as he is still not meeting the targets; fasting PG 7.5 mmol/l, HbA1c 10.2%?

*Comment*

He has improved significantly in a short period of time. His fasting PG has dropped and is now near target, and his urine tests have improved. While his HbA1c remains high, this reflects glycaemic control over the last 2 months and, as metformin was started only 1 month ago, its full impact on HbA1c is not yet apparent. It would be sensible to leave the present therapy and repeat the blood tests in 6–8 weeks. If he then remains above target, the metformin dose should be increased.

### CASE VIGNETTE 3.3

A 74-year-old widow who lives alone is obese (BMI 35.6 kg/m²) and presented with newly diagnosed diabetes, random PG 12.2 mmol/l, HbA1c 9.8%. When metformin was started, she developed diarrhoea and was unable to tolerate even low doses. Now 3 months after diagnosis, her control is not ideal with fasting PG 9.7 mmol/l and HbA1c 9.2%. What do I do next?

*Comment*

This lady is markedly overweight and is likely to have significant insulin resistance, so a thiazolidinedione (TZD, 'glitazone') would be logically appropriate as it would improve insulin sensitivity, though it does tend to increase weight. In the UK, these drugs are licensed for monotherapy. The current UK National Institute for Clinical Excellence (NICE) guidelines, however, recommend treatment with standard sulphonylurea therapy before starting a thiazolidinedione.

The treatment of choice in this lady would probably be a 'glitazone' such as rosiglitazone 4 mg daily or pioglitazone 15–30 mg daily. If this is not available or contraindicated, for example by cardiac failure, a sulphonylurea such as gliclazide 40–80 mg once daily would be best. It is preferable to avoid the very long-acting glibenclamide in this age group and in those who live alone as the risk of hypoglycaemia is substantial.

She also needs to be advised to control her food intake as weight gain is a common side effect of sulphonylurea or TZD treatment. Whichever drug is used, the dose may need to be adjusted depending upon her monitoring results – maximal doses are rosiglitazone 8 mg/24 hours, pioglitazone 45 mg/24 hours and gliclazide 160 mg b.d. or its equivalent, gliclazide modified release 120 mg daily.

## DIETARY AND LIFESTYLE CHANGES

### 3.13  What simple dietary advice should be given initially?

People newly diagnosed with diabetes are often unable to absorb all the new information given to them, and a few simple guides are useful (*Box 3.3*) until they can receive formal dietetic advice. Further questions on diet are discussed in Chapter 4.

---

**BOX 3.3  First steps to healthy eating for people with newly diagnosed diabetes**

- Do not add sugar to any food or drink – use artificial sweeteners if necessary
- Avoid all sweetened drinks and fruit juices – use low calorie, no added sugar or 'diet' drinks and squashes
- Do not eat sugary puddings or desserts, tinned fruit in syrup, tinned milk puddings or jellies – have fresh fruit
- Avoid all sweets, chocolate, cakes and sweet biscuits – if hungry between meals, eat fresh fruit
- Reduce fat in the diet

---

### 3.14  What exercise advice should be given at this stage?

Exercise should be discouraged while the patient is actively symptomatic and markedly hyperglycaemic (BG >15 mmol/l). The patient will only become excessively tired and demoralised. Once the BG is below this level, all patients should be encouraged to increase activity gradually, both in terms of formal exercise and normal physical activities.

More detailed exercise questions are discussed in Chapter 4.

### 3.15 What about self-monitoring in the initial stages of type 2 diabetes?

No absolute rules are appropriate. For patients on diet/lifestyle and on metformin alone there is no major requirement to test though many patients will wish to do so. Testing does, however, need a purpose – blood tests are both relatively expensive and uncomfortable.

The issue of testing in the longer term and the evidence for its value are dealt with in Chapter 11. Type 1 diabetes is an entirely different issue where some form of monitoring is almost always essential for safe outpatient management of newly diagnosed patients.

## PROBLEMS AFTER DIAGNOSIS

### 3.16 A week after initiating treatment, the patient is complaining bitterly of deteriorating vision? What should I do?

Many patients with newly diagnosed diabetes have marked fluctuations in visual acuity (VA) soon after treatment is started. This commonly happens when the initial PG levels were high (>20 mmol/l). The osmotic effect of chronic hyperglycaemia leads to a slow change in the refractive properties of the ocular lens. When PG levels fall, the process reverses fairly quickly, causing changing VA. Occasionally the astute optometrist who recognises the characteristic symptoms diagnoses diabetes. A good patient explanation is that the lens, as in a camera, has become swollen because of the high glucose and no longer focuses on the film. Only when the glucose has fallen and the lens has slowly shrunk to its usual size will it focus properly again.

However in type 2 diabetes retinopathy can be present at diagnosis. It is important to examine the retina carefully through dilated pupils with an ophthalmoscope, or by undertaking a retinal photograph to make sure retinopathy is not the cause. Once excluded, the patient can be reassured that the problems with their blurred vision will settle in the next 2–3 weeks. It is wise to advise newly diagnosed diabetic patients to delay changing their glasses for about 6–8 weeks, as subtle changes in VA are common over this time (*see also Ch. 15*).

### 3.17 Shortly after diagnosis of diabetes, the patient refuses to see me and won't speak to me on the phone. What should I do?

As with many other illnesses, it is easy to underestimate the impact of diabetes. There is often denial, anger and fear – the last when there is previous experience of diabetes in family or friends, especially where serious complications have occurred.

Management is not specific to diabetes, though a few points are:

■ Support from other family members is crucially important, especially with self-testing and remembering medication.

■ It is unhelpful to say: 'It's only mild diabetes, it only needs a change of diet'. There is no variety of diabetes that is mild! Most patients regard the condition as serious, and we need to sympathise and understand this.

■ A few patients will continue to deny the diagnosis and avoid treatment – some will need psychological assessment and help, which is often not easily available.

## OTHER ASPECTS OF LIFESTYLE

### 3.18 How long should I persist with diet and lifestyle changes alone?

A substantial number of patients will be controlled on diet and lifestyle measures alone, especially those with lower initial BG and HbA1c, for example pre-treatment fasting BGs of 7–12 mmol/l or HbA1c 7–9%. An example of a patient treated by diet and exercise alone is shown in *Table 3.2* (note the slow initial fall in HbA1c and the relatively limited weight loss). Improvement continues over the 6 months, and may continue thereafter. Some reasonable general principles are:

■ Significant *persisting* hyperglycaemic symptoms need intervention.

■ Continue with diet/lifestyle measures while there is continuing benefit, and as long as there are no major symptoms.

■ Add an OHA if glycaemic targets are then not met (*see Fig. 3.1*).

■ Final decisions on lipid interventions and the presence of microalbuminuria may need to wait until glycaemic control has been improved as much as practicable.

■ Sometimes short-term OHAs can produce an improvement which can subsequently be maintained by lifestyle changes alone.

| TABLE 3.2 Type 2 diabetes treated by diet and exercise alone | | | |
|---|---|---|---|
| | Fasting blood glucose (mmol/l) | Weight (kg) | HbA1c (%) |
| Diagnosis | 10.3 | 112.4 | 8.9 |
| + 6 weeks | 8.6 | 109.9 | 8.2 |
| + 12 weeks | 7.0 | 106.5 | 6.9 |
| + 6 months | 6.3 | 104.6 | 6.4 |

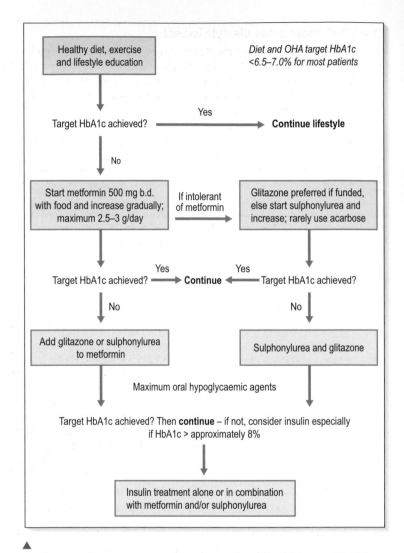

**Fig. 3.1** Outline management for overweight and obese patients. OHA, oral hypoglycaemic agent.

## 3.19  What about other lifestyle issues?

A full history should include other issues of importance, in particular smoking and alcohol. Other vascular risk factors should be assessed but it is not usually possible to fully assess these until diabetes has been controlled – both lipids and microalbuminuria are affected by poor glycaemic control and may improve once control is optimised.

Smoking should be firmly discouraged but it is often too stressful a time to attempt giving up immediately – this should usually be deferred until the patient is motivated to consider cessation (*see Appendices 1 and 2*).

Alcohol consumption should be assessed and reduction advised if above sensible drinking recommendations (*see Q. 4.28*) – many patients expect an absolute ban and are relieved!

## 3.20  Can initial management be summarised simply?

Hard to do, but general management principles are outlined in *Box 3.4*.

---

**BOX 3.4  General management principles of the management of type 2 diabetes**

- All newly diagnosed people with diabetes need to receive education – a diabetes nurse specialist and dietitian are usually the most effective educators.
- Over 85–95% of people with type 2 diabetes are overweight – weight loss is an important part of management. Metformin is then the oral agent of first choice (*Fig. 3.1*).
- Lean people (BMI < 24–25 kg/m² in Europeans) with type 2 diabetes are usually started on a sulphonylurea as initial treatment.
- Many people with type 2 diabetes should be encouraged to monitor their treatment by undertaking either blood or urine testing.
- Response to dietary treatment is usually seen within 4–8 weeks but an oral hypoglycaemic agent may need to be commenced earlier if the patient remains symptomatic. Diet and lifestyle measures may continue as long as weight is falling and exercise increasing, sometimes for over 6 months.
- Assessment of glycaemic control (HbA1c) should be undertaken at least every 6 months, or more frequently initially or if control is unsatisfactory.
- Annual screening is required to detect the complications of diabetes (eyes, kidneys, feet), starting at the time of diagnosis.
- Annual assessment is also required for cardiovascular risk factors (blood pressure, lipids, smoking, exercise), beginning soon after diagnosis.

# Dietary and lifestyle management

# 4

## SMOKING AND ALCOHOL

## PQ PATIENT QUESTIONS

## DIETARY MANAGEMENT

### 4.1    What is a diet trying to achieve?

A single diet may not be appropriate to all, but there are several overall aims for the majority of people with type 2 diabetes:

■ Weight loss
■ Improvement of glycaemic control
■ Improvement in cardiac risk factors and potential outcomes.

The same quality diet may obtain all three targets or fail to achieve weight loss simply because the calorie content is too high. A dietetic referral and assessment needs to include each of these aims if it is to be effective, while also sensitive to the culture, finances and lifestyle of the individual.

Increasing the proportion of vegetables, fruit, nuts and oily fish in the diet and following other features of the Mediterranean diet (e.g. small amounts of lean meat, whole grains) are helpful in improving cardiovascular outcomes for people with diabetes as well as those without.[1–4]

### 4.2    Is there a simple model for explaining a balanced meal?

The plate model for balancing food portions is one useful, though limited, concept. When putting a main meal on a plate, the meat portion should fill less than a quarter of the plate. The remaining part should be divided roughly in half, one part filled with vegetables and the other with starchy food.

In some countries, food 'pyramids' are used to explain the ideal balance between foods. The pyramid base includes grains, beans and starchy foods with 5–6 servings per day recommended, while at the top are fats, sweets and alcohol, to be eaten only occasionally. In between are vegetables (3–5 servings) and fruit (2–4 servings) with dairy foods and meat (2–3 servings). Recent suggested revisions have emphasised more vegetables, legumes, vegetable oils and nuts, and reduced the recommended fruit, starch and meat components. These recommendations provide generous total servings and so should only be used by experienced dietitians who can also emphasise portion size control (see the American Diabetes Association website *www.diabetes.org/main/health/nutrition*).

### 4.3    The dietitian has told my patient they can eat sugar, but surely people with diabetes should have a sugar-free diet?

The modern approach is not to ban sugar entirely as this is often unpalatable, but to allow a small amount, preferably mixed with other foods and not taken on an empty stomach. This makes sense when we understand that the glycaemic index of sugar (sucrose) is in fact lower than white bread. Sugar is a disaccharide, and when digested releases equal quantities of glucose and fructose. The latter monosaccharide does not affect plasma glucose (PG) levels and is found commonly in fruit giving a sweet taste. Compare this to the polysaccharide starch in white bread: when this is digested, all the energy released is as glucose and leads to rapidly rising PG levels.

Allowing patients some sugar is acceptable but the total quantity should be kept reasonably small since sugar is high in calories and will contribute to weight gain. In addition, the aim is to change a person's preference from sweet-tasting foods.

If sugary foods are to be taken as a treat or part of the diet, it is best to consume them as part of or at the end of a meal. This means that the sugar content will be less rapidly digested and the effect on PG levels reduced.

## 4.4 What are the common misconceptions about diet in type 2 diabetes?

These are many and various; some are shown in *Table 4.1*. It is also true that the evidence on which dietary principles are based is not as good as it should be, and that many 'special diets' have not been adequately tested or compared, especially in long-term use.

**TABLE 4.1 Common misconceptions about diabetes and dietary advice**

| Misconception | Explanation |
| --- | --- |
| People with diabetes need a special diet, different from the rest of the family | People with diabetes are advised to follow healthy eating principles which would be good for all family members |
| Starchy foods can be eaten as much as necessary to satisfy the appetite | Eating starchy foods to satisfy the appetite will often lead to weight gain. Starchy foods need to be kept to reasonable portion sizes |
| If my test results are high, all starchy foods need to be cut out or severely reduced | Everyone needs a balanced diet with some starchy foods. If tests remain high with a balanced diet, diabetes treatment may need adjustment |
| Fat intake has no effect on diabetic control | Fats are high in calories – liberal intake of fats will tend to lead to weight gain and increasing insulin resistance |
| Olive oil and sunflower oil are good for you so you can have as much as you like | These types of oil are preferable to animal fats but high intake will lead to a large calorie intake and weight gain. They should be used in moderation |

**TABLE 4.1  (*Cont'd*) Common misconceptions about diabetes and dietary advice**

| Misconception | Explanation |
|---|---|
| I have been recommended to take five pieces of fruit and five portions vegetables per day | The recommendation is five portions of fruit *and* vegetables per day. If weight reduction is required, five pieces of fruit may be too large a calorie intake, especially if taken as well as meals |
| All my favourite recipes have to be thrown out now I have diabetes | Many recipes can be adapted to fit into a healthy eating diabetes diet |
| A tin of baked beans contains sugar so is not allowed | The amount of sugar in a portion of baked beans is small and is acceptable. Baked beans are a good source of carbohydrate as, like other pulses, they contain soluble fibre and have a low glycaemic index |
| Meat doesn't need to be counted as it doesn't contain carbohydrate | Meat is a source of protein and fat with a high calorie content. Most people eat too-large portions of meat; 50–75 g of lean cooked meat is sufficient, approximately the size of a pack of cards |
| Brown bread is better than white | Brown bread or wholemeal is no better than white bread; whole-grain is the preferred choice |

## 4.5    What is the glycaemic index?

When food containing carbohydrate is eaten and digested, glucose is released and absorbed into the blood stream (*see Q. 1.2*), which increases PG levels. Different types of carbohydrate-containing food release glucose and affect PG levels in a variable way (*Fig. 4.1*). Thus a glucose drink results in PG levels rising rapidly and, in a person without diabetes, falling fairly quickly as insulin is released from the pancreas. At the other end of the spectrum, eating an apple results in a much slower rise in the PG level as the digestive process takes time to release the glucose.[5,6]

In people with diabetes, the pancreas is unable to respond to a rapidly rising PG level and the treatments for type 2 diabetes do not fully correct this problem. Hence people with diabetes are encouraged to follow a diet low in simple sugars. The term 'glycaemic index' (GI) has been coined to describe the rise in PG levels after consuming a carbohydrate-containing food. It relates not only to the peak level but also to the area under the curve for the 2-hour period after food is consumed. A GI of 100 refers to the response to 50 g glucose or white bread in a normal person without diabetes. All other foods with an equivalent carbohydrate value are measured against this standard (e.g. the GI of an apple is 52).[6]

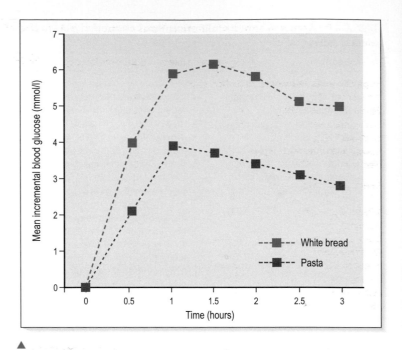

**Fig. 4.1** The mean rise in blood glucose after different foods, used to calculate glycaemic index by comparison with glucose.

### 4.6 Why is the glycaemic index of similar carbohydrate-containing food so variable?

The variation is due to the speed at which food is digested and glucose released into the gut and so available for absorption into the blood stream. White bread contains little fibre and the starch is available for rapid digestion by gut enzymes, whereas in whole-grain bread (*not wholemeal*), the starch is in the cereal grains, which need to be digested before the glucose can be released. These types of bread result in a much slower rise in PG levels. Wholemeal breads have a high GI as, in the processing of the flour, the grains are disrupted releasing the starch for rapid digestion. People with diabetes will benefit from taking low GI foods, as their PG levels will demonstrate fewer fluctuations which are difficult to control with existing treatments.

Glycaemic indices of foods also vary according to how they are prepared and with which other foods they are served. For instance, addition of fat to the food generally delays gastric emptying and digestion of the starch

**TABLE 4.2  Glycaemic index of different types of cooked potato and of some common foods**

|  | Glycaemic index | Carbohydrate (g) | Fat (g) |
|---|---|---|---|
| **Type of potato and average portion size** | | | |
| Plain crisps 50 g | 54 | 24 | 16 |
| Mashed potatoes 120 g | 91 | 16 | 0 |
| Boiled unpeeled new potatoes 175 g | 65 | 21 | 0 |
| Baked potato, no fat 120 g | 93 | 15 | 0 |
| Fine-cut chips 120 g | 75 | 49 | 26 |
| **Common foods** (*GI only*) | | | |
| White bread | 100 | | |
| Wholemeal bread | 100 | | |
| Porridge | 87 | | |
| Cornflakes cereal | 119 | | |
| All Bran cereal | 42 | | |
| Baked beans | 69 | | |
| Watermelon | 72 | | |
| Full fat milk | 27 | | |
| Digestive biscuits | 84 | | |
| Sucrose | 83 | | |

leading to a lower GI. There are also some problems with how the GI reflects whole foods (*Table 4.2*).

## 4.7   Does increasing the proportion of low glycaemic index foods improve diabetic control?

Some trials have shown that increasing the proportion of low GI foods in the diet led to an improvement in HbA1c.[6] Additionally, when low GI foods are taken as part of a weight-reducing diet, satiety has been improved compared to high GI foods. This is obviously important in people with type 2 diabetes where weight reduction is commonly needed.

## 4.8   What about 'ethnic' and 'Mediterranean' diets?

It is essential that dietary advice be both practicable and culturally and financially acceptable to the individual, the cook and the family. This requires skilled dietitians who are aware of, and experienced in, the eating habits of the local population cultures. Many such cultures had naturally extremely healthy patterns, which have now been damaged by westernisation and easy availability of pre-prepared, high-fat food in abundance. A detailed consideration of these issues is beyond this book, but all health professionals should be aware of relevant local issues (e.g. the high-fat content of some Indo-Asian diets).

Mediterranean diets are also associated with improved survival and reduced macrovascular outcomes, both in the general population and in patients with cardiac disease.[3,4] There does not appear to be a single dietary ingredient (e.g. olive oil or red wine) responsible for this! In other studies high fish consumption has been associated with decreased mortality.

### 4.9 My patient with type 1 diabetes has talked about a DAFNE diet course for helping her control. What is she talking about?

DAFNE stands for 'dietary adjustment for normal eating'.[7] This is a German-originating model of dietary therapy for type 1 diabetes where patients go on a course to learn the effects of different meals on their post-prandial glucoses and to learn to calculate/estimate the short-acting insulin dose needed. It has recently been adopted by a few centres in the UK and is being trialled under the auspices of Diabetes UK. Its advantages are that it allows more natural eating with patient-controlled adjustment of insulin and, in trials thus far, has shown improved glycaemic control (see the Diabetes UK website *www.diabetes.org.uk* for more details).

## WEIGHT LOSS

### 4.10 What are the benefits of weight loss on other health aspects?

A relatively small degree of weight loss can have major benefits in many areas.[8,9] For example, a 10% weight reduction in someone starting at 100 kg is estimated to produce:
- significant falls in systolic and diastolic BP
- a 10% reduction in total cholesterol
- a 20–25% fall in total mortality
- a 30–40% reduction in diabetes-related deaths.[8]

### 4.11 Why is weight loss so difficult in people with diabetes?

For the same reasons as people without diabetes – they continue to eat and drink more calories than their body requires for their lifestyle. This is often difficult for the patient to admit and many will tell you how little they eat. As people get older there is a tendency to gain weight as the same quantity of food is consumed but metabolic rate decreases as less exercise or activity is undertaken. Appetite responds slowly to the body's requirement and is often driven by habit rather than need.

Getting the patient motivated to want to lose weight is the first step. Dietitian referral can be helpful and a sensible weight-reducing eating plan devised, but it is not a panacea. Some patients need help with weight-reducing medication (*see Q. 4.12*).

### 4.12 Are weight-reducing drugs or surgical techniques of value?

*Weight-reducing drugs*

The main current drugs are orlistat and sibutramine.

■ *Orlistat* is a pancreatic lipase inhibitor which works by reducing absorption of dietary fat. Consequently, its main side effect is flatulence and liquid oily stools.

■ *Sibutramine* is a centrally acting appetite suppressant. Use in diabetes needs to be carefully considered since it can cause a significant rise in BP, and is not recommended in those with pre-existing hypertension.

These drugs are expensive and in trials have been effective only when used in a well-structured, weight-reduction programme. The National Institute for Clinical Excellence (NICE) guidelines recommend these drugs be used when there is evidence of initial weight loss by dietary restriction alone (*see www.nice.org.uk*).

Antidepressants such as fluoxetine can be successful in some patients where low mood makes following a strict weight-reducing diet difficult.

All these drugs need careful use – consult the *BNF* and datasheets.

*Surgical techniques*

There are surgical techniques such as gastric banding for the treatment of obesity. In the UK and elsewhere, there is relatively limited availability. NICE guidelines suggest this might be considered for a person with type 2 diabetes with BMI >35 kg/m$^2$ after all other methods of weight loss have been tried, but they appear to have considerable promise in patients with morbid obesity and the associated problems.

### EXERCISE AND TYPE 2 DIABETES

### 4.13 What is the evidence that exercise is beneficial in glycaemic control?

There is substantial evidence that adequate amounts of exercise improve glycaemic control, but it would be wrong to limit the benefits just to glucose. Studies have shown that exercise can produce multiple benefits in global health terms, particularly in cardiovascular terms, though at differing intensities:[10,11]

■ *Diabetes and obesity*: lower HbA1c and PG levels; reduced abdominal circumference

■ *Cardiovascular health*: improved lipid profile; reduced BP; increased aerobic fitness; increased lifespan

■ *General*: increased energy level; sleeping better; improved mood

### 4.14 How much exercise is necessary to produce benefit?

Exercise is difficult to measure and prone to over-reporting! It appears that there is a continuum of benefit with some improvements at the lower end of the scale, but some only achievable with frequent, substantial exercise.

One formal recommendation is to encourage inactive individuals to take 30 minutes of exercise on most days of the week, while those already active should try to incorporate more vigorous exercise at least three times weekly.

Additionally, further minor exercise should be encouraged whenever there is the opportunity, for example:

- climbing stairs rather than using lifts
- walking rather than using the car for short errands
- parking further away from work, the shops, etc.
- walking one or two stops before/after catching the bus
- doing more gardening.

There is conflicting evidence about 'snack-tivity', multiple shorter periods of activity. Most authorities regard it as better than nothing, but not the equivalent of a single summed period of exercise.

'Step-meters' are used by some as a way of measuring and encouraging increased activity.

### 4.15 How can I quantitate and compare exercise levels?

One scale is the METs: 1 MET is equivalent to the resting metabolic rate. METs values for various types of exercise are shown in *Table 4.3*.

### 4.16 How can I persuade people to increase their exercise levels?

As with any other lifestyle modification, individuals have to be motivated and prepared to change (*see Appendix 1*). There is some evidence to back the use of 'green prescriptions' where GPs in New Zealand provide a formal prescription for treatment by exercise, with the local sports organisation then contacting the patient.

### 4.17 Why does exercise lead to high glucose levels on some occasions and to hypoglycaemia on others?

The effect of exercise on blood glucose (BG) levels is complex.[12] The response to a short burst of vigorous exercise depends on the prevailing BG and insulin levels. Exercise is accompanied by secretion of stress hormones, catecholamines, cortisol, glucagon and growth hormone. These alone lead to a rise in BG concentration. However, if prevailing insulin levels are relatively high and the BG levels are normal, glucose is driven into cells, thus lowering BG concentrations. The balance between these two effects is the reason why response to exercise is variable. In addition, in a person without diabetes, exercise tends to reduce pancreatic insulin secretion,

TABLE 4.3 METs values for various types of exercise

| Exercise | METs value* |
|---|---|
| Desk work, driving, fishing | ~1.5 |
| Standing | 2 |
| Walking at 2 mph (3 kph) | 2 |
| Housework | 2.5 |
| Cycling flat at 5 mph (8 kph) | 3 |
| Gardening | 3 |
| Lawn-mowing | 3 |
| Walking at 4 mph (6.5 kph) | 4 |
| Swimming slowly | 4 |
| Slow dancing | 4 |
| Golf (with no cart!) | 4 |
| Badminton/tennis | 5 |
| Cycling flat at 10 mph (16 kph) | 6 |
| Fast step dancing | 6 |
| Jogging at 5–10 mph (8–16 kph) | 8–16 |
| Downhill skiing | 8 |
| Cycling at 16 mph (25 kph) | 9 |
| Cross-country skiing | 12 |

* All values are approximate. kph, kilometres per hour; mph, miles per hour.

whereas in diabetic patients insulin levels are unaffected as insulin absorption from the subcutaneous depot continues or sulphonylurea action continues to stimulate pancreatic insulin secretion.

If BG is high (>8 mmol/l) at the beginning of exercise and insulin levels are relatively low, the stress hormone effect leads to rising BG concentrations. If BG levels are well controlled (4–6 mmol/l) and the patient has reasonable levels of insulin in the circulation, vigorous exercise will tend to lower the glucose as the insulin drives it into the cells, over-riding the stress hormone effects. This variable response can lead to intense frustration for many patients. Understanding the critical factors involved in exercise can be helpful. Glucose levels can affect performance in competitive sport; high BG levels and under-insulinisation result in fatigue and under-performance.

## 4.18 How does exercise lead to hypoglycaemia many hours later?

During exercise, stored glucose is released from muscles and utilised to complete the activity. Later, the body needs to replace the glucose stores in muscle and this occurs over a period of hours. During this time, glucose uptake in the periphery is much higher than normal and BG concentrations may fall if adequate compensatory carbohydrate is omitted. Thus, it is unusual for a patient to become hypoglycaemic during a game of squash, tennis, soccer or rugby while the later part of an 18-hole round of golf or an all-day cricket game are more likely scenarios. Other common causes are skiing, energetic walking, a day out sailing or a busy day's gardening.

For the shorter duration sports, the commonest time for hypoglycaemia to occur is between 3 and 12 hours later, but for longer activities or evening sport, it may even extend to the following morning. For patients on insulin, a reduction in dose before the anticipated exercise is advisable, and certainly a reduced evening or bedtime dose if the exercise is in the afternoon or evening. The same may be true for patients taking sulphonylureas alone or in combination. There should be no hypoglycaemia while taking metformin or 'glitazones' alone, though BG levels will tend to run at lower levels than they would in the absence of exercise. Some patients are aware of this fall in glucose levels and may feel hypoglycaemic symptoms even though BG does not drop below 4 mmol/l.

---

### 4.19 What are the principles behind management of diabetes and exercise?

In brief, these can be summarized as:
- Exercise usually produces an immediate short-term rise in BG followed by a longer-term fall.
- The greatest risk of hypoglycaemia is later after the exercise (often that evening) and up to 12–16 hours afterwards.
- Appropriate treatment for hypoglycaemia should be readily available at all times.
- Predictable exercise usually requires a reduction in insulin doses before and for some hours afterwards. For well-controlled patients on sulphonylureas, doses may need to be reduced or omitted.
- The heavier and longer the exercise, the greater the reduction will need to be (most often 10–40%, but can be more).
- On a skiing or similar active holiday, insulin doses or sulphonylurea drugs should be reduced by 25–40% from the first day for the duration of the holiday.
- An alternative approach is to have extra carbohydrate following exercise, but often both extra food and reduction in insulin dose are needed.
- For overweight patients, it is preferable to reduce insulin/oral agents rather than to have to eat extra during and after sport.
- Response to exercise affects individual patients differently.
- Patients need to monitor and record their BG levels frequently before, during and after exercise when they are learning how to manage their diabetes.
- Health care professionals need to encourage patients to discuss the management of diabetes and exercise and review monitoring results together.

## SMOKING AND ALCOHOL

### 4.20   Is smoking as important a risk factor in people with diabetes as in others?

This is a harder question to answer than might be expected. Most of the evidence on smoking comes from subgroup analysis of larger studies involving people without diabetes or observational studies and, understandably, none from controlled trials. The effect of smoking on glycaemic control is uncertain.[13]

*Microvascular complications*
Most studies in diabetic populations have found smoking to be associated with increased development and progression of nephropathy and neuropathy, often two- to three-fold, but not so clearly with retinopathy. For macrovascular disease the relative risk (RR) is around 1.5–2 in most studies, but with evidence that it may take longer for the effect of previous smoking to wear off than in non-diabetic individuals. Smoking cessation is therefore extremely important as this is an avoidable risk: normal cessation models appear to be effective though depression may be more prevalent and affect success rates[13] (*see Appendix 2*).

*Macrovascular disease*
Smoking appears to have just as adverse an effect on cardiovascular disease in people with diabetes and, as it represents an additional risk, some studies such as MRFIT imply even worse outcomes.[14] Smoking habits should be assessed regularly – too often this is not routinely documented and ex-smokers return to the habit without their medical team realising: the patient is unlikely to volunteer the information! Relapse rates after 1 year off smoking are around 20–40%.

### 4.21   How should smoking be managed?

Everyone with diabetes who smokes should be advised to stop, though they may not yet be ready to accept the advice or to act upon it. Once again their willingness to change should be assessed and support offered in a non-confrontational way (*see Appendices 1 and 2*).

There is no evidence that people with diabetes differ from the general population in their response to individual or group advice.[13,15]

#### 4.22 Can pharmacological aids to stopping smoking be used in diabetes?

Yes. Nicotine replacement therapy is first-line treatment as in the general population for smokers of over 15 cigarettes daily, increasing the rate of quitting by 50–100%.

Bupropion is also effective but a limited maximal dose is advised in people on insulin or secretagogues as there is thought to be a greater risk of seizure with hypoglycaemia. This should not logically apply in obese type 2 patients on diet or metformin alone, but no data are currently available. The usual exclusions and advice on its use apply.

 **PATIENT QUESTIONS**

#### 4.23 Why does my blood sugar go up when I eat a meal with no sugar in it?

Starchy foods such as bread, potatoes and pasta when digested in the stomach release energy in the form of glucose. This will be absorbed through the stomach wall and lead to a rise in your blood glucose level. The body relies on sugar as its main source of energy so we all need some starchy foods in our diet. If your blood glucose levels are rising too high, it may be that your diabetes treatment needs adjustment.

#### 4.24 Can artificial sweeteners be used?

Yes. These are safe in all reasonable quantities. The perceived difference in taste between these and sucrose often appears to diminish when sucrose is excluded, though the powdered versions are usually less appreciated. It is, however, advisable to try to change away from sweeter foods, and a gradual slow reduction in sugar/sweeteners is often achievable.

#### 4.25 Are 'commercial' diets (e.g. Weight Watchers, Jenny Craig, Atkins) suitable for people with diabetes?

There is little scientific evidence about most of these diets in diabetes and often health care professionals have been against them. Several studies have recently shown that they may be effective in producing weight loss in the short-term, but unfortunately the initial rapid weight loss often fails to be maintained. Most doctors would now permit many of their patients with type 2 diabetes to undertake such diets *under the supervision of an experienced dietitian*, but with the proviso that a long-term dietary plan will then be agreed and followed. Some of these diets (e.g. Atkins) require some vitamin or mineral supplementation, and may also require reduction in diabetes tablets or insulin.

The Atkins diet, which relies on ketogenesis, is not recommended for people with type 1 diabetes.

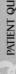
PATIENT QUESTIONS

### 4.26  What sort of exercise is most beneficial?

The best forms are those that make you slightly breathless and quicken your pulse, such as fast walking, cycling, the gym or swimming. Resistance training using low weights and multiple repetitions is a useful alternative for those with mobility limitations (e.g. arthritis, stroke, claustrophobia, etc.).

Most important is a form of exercise that you will enjoy or, at least, persist with. So involve others (family or friends) and go walking, consider joining a group activity such as church or community-based classes or dance lessons. These will be enjoyable, sociable and good for many aspects of your health, not just the diabetes.

### 4.27  How will diabetes affect sporting activity?

Exercise is beneficial for people with type 2 diabetes, promoting weight loss, a reduction in vascular risk and a sense of well-being. There are few major sports which represent a major problem, except possibly rock climbing and scuba diving, where the consequences of hypoglycaemia would be severe. These are really only an issue for those on insulin, and even scuba diving is now permitted under strict conditions for those with excellent glycaemic control.

Good education, careful blood glucose self-monitoring and recording with consideration of the timing of exercise, will normally allow patients to determine the effect of activity on blood glucose levels and allow the development of appropriate strategies. Some patients require support and encouragement by their physicians and/or educators. A few competitive sportsmen or women will require expert help, but it is worth remembering that people with diabetes are well represented among Olympic and world-class athletes in many sports.

### 4.28  What about alcohol consumption?

There are several issues with this question, and controversy still surrounds some of them.[16,17] However, it is no longer appropriate to ban alcohol for patients with diabetes (as happened previously).

■ *Healthy drinking limits*: These are the same as for patients without diabetes – a limit of two standard drinks per day for women, three for men. People with diabetes should be advised not to miss food because of the alcohol, even though the calorific value of the beer, wine or spirits has to be taken into account. The risk of hypoglycaemia appears to be increased if food is omitted, while hypoglycaemia and drunkenness are easily confused. It is sensible to advise people with insulin-treated diabetes to make sure they take alcohol with a meal or snack.

■ *Health benefits of alcohol*: These are still debated but are consistent over many studies: it does appear clear that moderate drinking is associated with improved cardiovascular outcomes. But experts do not recommend taking up drinking specifically for this purpose!

■ *Which alcohol?*: The previous evidence favouring red wine specifically is no longer clear cut, and it appears likely that alcohol itself has a role. Sweet wines and heavier beers are clearly a dietary calorie issue, but most low alcohol beers are also a problem as they substitute assorted carbohydrates for the missing alcohol.

■ *Drinking and driving*: In patients at risk of hypoglycaemia, the possible potentiation by alcohol and the confusion between hypoglycaemia and intoxication make the only sensible advice: 'Don't drink and drive'.

# Use of oral hypoglycaemic agents

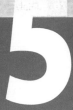

## WHEN TO START AN ORAL AGENT

### 5.1    When should an oral hypoglycaemic agent be started?

*Figure 3.1* shows the approach to glucose management in type 2 diabetes. First-line therapy should nearly always be dietary and lifestyle – the patient should not receive the message that the major treatment is tablets! In the UKPDS, dietary therapy was the sole intervention for the first 3 months and achieved a mean 2% reduction in HbA1c, more than that achieved by any single oral hypoglycaemic agent (OHA). Most of the latter will produce mean reductions of 1.0–1.5% in HbA1c, except for acarbose which is much less effective.

When the initial plasma glucose (PG) level is high, many clinicians are tempted to commence an OHA at diagnosis. Unless patients are highly symptomatic it is usually better to start with diet and exercise alone, except if there are important personal indications (e.g. forthcoming exams or foreign travel). People with newly diagnosed diabetes have often been drinking large quantities of sugary drinks such as lemonade, 'Coke' or fruit juices to quench their thirst. Just removing these and other simple sugars from the diet often leads to a rapid fall in PG and control of the symptoms. The consequent improvement demonstrates to the patient the importance of diet in diabetes treatment.

In general those patients with higher PG levels at diagnosis (once simple sugars are removed) are more likely to need OHAs in addition to diet. If there is concern about the initial PG level, it is prudent to review the patient in a few days to monitor their response and reassess the need for medication. If a sulphonylurea in particular is prescribed too early, some patients will develop problems with hypoglycaemia and weight gain within the first few weeks of treatment.

Usually use of an OHA is delayed until lifestyle measures alone have proved unsuccessful in achieving adequate control after a reasonable trial (*see Q. 3.18*). This will depend on the 'target' level of control that is desired, which may obviously be lower in HbA1c terms for some patients than for others, such as the elderly living alone. There is no hard evidence to base this on, but some data suggest that optimal control needs to be achieved within the first 6–12 months, as people frequently ' track' at that level thereafter.

**TABLE 5.1  Current drug treatment options in diabetes**

| Function | Name | Action |
|---|---|---|
| Drugs decreasing insulin resistance[1–5] | Metformin | Biguanide, detailed mechanism unclear |
| | Thiazolidinediones (TZDs, 'glitazones') | Work via PPAR-gamma receptors |
| Drugs increasing insulin secretion[6–9] | Sulphonylureas | Stimulate insulin secretion, mainly second phase |
| | Meglitinides | Stimulate insulin secretion, mainly first phase |
| Drugs reducing carbohydrate absorption[10,11] | Acarbose | Inhibitor of intestinal alpha-glucosidase |

## 5.2    What are the current options?

Despite some recent advances, there are still relatively few options, and the thiazolidinediones (TZDs) and meglitinides currently have restrictions on their usage (*Table 5.1*).

## 5.3    On what basis should I choose the initial oral agent?

Weight! Perhaps 85–95% of newly diagnosed patients with type 2 diabetes in Western countries are overweight or obese and have some or many components of the metabolic syndrome (*see Q. 1.12*). In these patients metformin is the drug of choice – sulphonylureas are now rarely the drug of first choice (*see also Case vignettes 5.1–5.3*).

The evidence for this is largely based on the UKPDS, where the obese group treated with metformin produced a much greater reduction in events than the main intensive group treated with sulphonylureas or insulin (*see Fig. 2.3*).[12]

A summary of the main agents available is shown in *Table 5.2*.

## USING METFORMIN

## 5.4    Why the recent change from sulphonylurea to metformin as a first-line oral agent for most patients?

The main reason is the clinical trial data, though increasing obesity and recognition of the metabolic syndrome also play a part. Metformin targets the main problem of insulin resistance, and in the UKPDS the obese group treated with metformin showed a much greater drop in vascular events than the sulphonylurea/insulin groups.[12]

**TABLE 5.2 Oral hypoglycaemic agents**

| Class of drug | Name | Action | Common side effects | Contraindications |
|---|---|---|---|---|
| Biguanide | Metformin | Reduces hepatic gluconeogenesis and increases peripheral glucose utilisation | Nausea, vomiting and diarrhoea | Renal failure (serum creatinine > 150 µmol/l) Liver impairment Heart failure |
| Sulphonylurea | Glibenclamide Gliclazide Glimepiride Glipizide Gliquidone (Chlorpropamide) (Tolbutamide) | Stimulates insulin secretion by the pancreas | Weight gain Hypoglycaemia | In renal impairment gliclazide, gliquidone and tolbutamide are safe but avoid glibenclamide and chlorpropamide, as hypoglycaemia can be a problem with drug accumulation |
| Meglitinide | Nateglinide Repaglinide | Stimulates insulin release | Hypoglycaemia | Renal or hepatic impairment Pregnancy |
| Thiazolidinedione | Pioglitazone Rosiglitazone | Increases insulin sensitivity | Fluid retention Weight gain Anaemia | Heart disease as can precipitate heart failure Hepatic or renal impairment |
| Alpha-glucosidase inhibitor | Acarbose | Inhibits intestinal alpha-glucosidase delaying absorption of starch and sucrose | Flatulence, abdominal distension and diarrhoea | Inflammatory bowel disease |

There are increasing numbers of combination tablets becoming available with two anti-diabetic agents of differing action. They offer the advantages of ease and probable improved adherence, but still await adequate long-term studies and should be used only when the doses are exactly what would otherwise be recommended. Examples are sulphonylurea/metformin, and metformin/rosiglitazone (Avandamet).

Metformin is not associated with weight gain whereas all other therapies are. What is not clear is the lowest level of BMI or waist circumference down to which metformin should be the first choice, or indeed if there is a lower limit.

## 5.5 What are the major side effects of metformin?

 The main drawback of metformin is the high incidence of gastrointestinal side effects of nausea and diarrhoea, together with flatulence, abdominal pain and a metallic taste. Loose bowel movements can be an intermittent rather than a continuous problem.

These effects are usually dose-related and transient so it is always worth starting at low dose (e.g. 500 mg b.d. with meals) and gradually increasing (e.g. to 1 g b.d.) after 2 weeks or so. It is sensible to warn all patients about these side effects; approximately 15–25% of patients will report some initial gastrointestinal problems if questioned and it seems to be a more frequent problem with women than with men. For some patients (around 5%), the side effects are so persistent and severe that metformin has to be withdrawn. However, many patients will tolerate the drug despite some side effects, and it is worth exploring with the patient the highest tolerable dose. Even low-dose metformin 500 mg once or twice daily is valuable and can obviously be used in combination with other OHAs and with insulin in type 2 diabetes. The recommended maximal dose is 2550 mg/day (850 mg × 3), though some clinicians go up to 3 g daily for very obese patients (e.g. > 100 kg).

Other less common side effects include lactic acidosis (*see Q. 9.11*) and decreased vitamin B12 absorption. A former biguanide – phenformin – was withdrawn some years ago because of the high risk of lactic acidosis.

## 5.6 How does metformin work?

Despite being in use for over 30 years, this still isn't fully known at molecular level. Metformin decreases gluconeogenesis and enhances peripheral glucose utilisation.[13]

## 5.7 When is metformin contraindicated?

 This is controversial, the anxiety being the very rare lactic acidosis which carries a high mortality. The official list is outlined in *Table 5.3*, but evidence for most of these restrictions is almost entirely lacking.[14] Despite wide

**TABLE 5.3 Contraindications to the use of metformin**

| Listed contraindication | Explanation/normal usage |
|---|---|
| Hepatic impairment | Clinical liver disease, not just increased liver function tests |
| Renal impairment | Serum creatinine over 130–150 μmol/l |
| Ketoacidosis | |
| Severe dehydration | |
| Shock | |
| Trauma | Withdraw immediately if acutely ill |
| Respiratory failure | |
| Severe peripheral vascular disease | |
| Recent myocardial infarction | |
| Heart failure | Only use if well controlled |
| Alcohol dependency | See hepatic impairment |
| Use of X-ray contrast media | Withdraw or use newer low-risk media |

increases in its use, problems are extremely rare even when the official recommendations have not been adhered to. While one cannot recommend its use against guidelines, there are occasions when it is the only useful agent and some fully informed patients will choose to take it (see discussion in a recent article by Jones et al[14]).

## 5.8 How is metformin best used in practice?

There are some simple rules for its best use:

- ■ *Always* start with low dose (e.g. 500 mg b.d.), then increase some weeks later.
- ■ Always take *during* a meal, never on an empty stomach.
- ■ Warn patients about possible gastrointestinal side effects, stressing that most are transient.
- ■ If side effects persist, halve the dose and then gradually increase more slowly; twice daily is often better for adherence than three times daily.
- ■ Emphasise that it will take some days to weeks to become effective.
- ■ For most patients a dose of 1 g b.d. should be the eventual target.
- ■ It can be combined with other agents (*see Q. 5.17*).

(*See Case vignettes 5.1–5.3.*)

## USING SULPHONYLUREAS AND MEGLITINIDES

## 5.9 How do sulphonylureas work?

Sulphonylureas increase pancreatic insulin secretion. This is done through a calcium channel mechanism, and induces an increase in both first- and second-phase insulin release.

## 5.10   What are the major side effects and contraindications for sulphonylureas?

Hypoglycaemia is the main issue with sulphonylureas, but is hardly a side effect! Weight gain is common. They are otherwise well tolerated with occasional effects of rashes, nausea, vomiting, diarrhoea and constipation. They may rarely cause hepatic problems including cholestatic jaundice and eventual liver failure, as well as blood dyscrasias and severe skin reactions.[7]

They should not be used in severe hepatic disease and only a few are safe in renal impairment (*see Q. 5.11*). They should be avoided while breast feeding and in patients with porphyria.

These agents should be used with caution, especially in the elderly, those frail or living alone and in patients with renal failure as severe protracted hypoglycaemia can occur, especially with glibenclamide and chlorpropamide.

## 5.11   How are sulphonylureas best used?

Some useful advice can be summarised:

- Start with a low dose and increase at about 2-weekly intervals unless BG levels are initially very high.
- Sulphonylureas require residual beta cell function in order to be effective.
- Some patients are very sensitive and need very small doses (e.g. glibenclamide or glipizide 2.5 mg daily, gliclazide 40 mg daily, gliclazide modified release 30 mg daily).
- Always warn and teach patients about hypoglycaemia.
- Weight gain in the first 3–6 months is to be expected, averaging around 3 kg.
- There is no benefit at all in exceeding maximum doses or using more than one sulphonylurea.
- Gliclazide, tolbutamide and gliquidone are the preferred agents in patients with renal impairment, but use with care.
- Severe hypoglycaemia with sulphonylureas is a medical emergency with a significant mortality and requires immediate hospital admission (*see Ch. 7*).

## 5.12   What is the difference with the newer agents like repaglinide?

The meglitinides (currently repaglinide and nateglinide) also stimulate insulin secretion but do so through a different mechanism and predominantly enhance *first-phase* insulin release, thus reducing immediate post-prandial hyperglycaemia.[8,9]

Had they been invented before sulphonylureas or were cheaper, they would probably be preferred as they cause less hypoglycaemia but are more expensive. Particular points are:

- Start with a small dose.
- Take up to 30 minutes before meals.
- No meal – no tablet!
- Side effects include gastrointestinal upsets and rashes as well as hypoglycaemia.

Case vignettes 5.1–5.3 illustrate circumstances in which a choice of OHAs can be made.

### CASE VIGNETTE 5.1

A sedentary man aged 55 years has had type 2 diabetes for 5 months, BMI has fallen from 32 to 31 kg/m² on diet and exercise alone. Results are now steady, with fasting glucose 8.1 mmol/l, HbA1c 7.4% and creatinine 72 μmol/l.

*Comment*

Glycaemic control is suboptimal and, 5 months later, this is probably the best he will achieve with diet alone. You could continue with diet alone if he was still losing weight but commonly patients fail to sustain their initial good results. Metformin 500 mg twice daily is the next step, and may need doubling thereafter.

### CASE VIGNETTE 5.2

A 68-year-old Afro-Caribbean woman was diagnosed on routine screening 8 months ago with a fasting BG of 9.8 mmol/l. Her BMI remains between 24 and 25 kg/m² on diet and exercise alone. The current fasting glucose is 7.7 mmol/l, HbA1c 6.9% and creatinine 64 μmol/l.

*Comment*

This patient has moderately good control but what is the appropriate target for a patient controlled by diet alone? The National Institute for Clinical Excellence (NICE) guidelines recommend a target for each person with diabetes in the range 6.5–7.5%, the decision to be made on individual circumstances. The UKPDS indicated that best outcomes in microvascular and macrovascular terms was in the group with lowest HbA1c: a mean of less than 6%. Thus, if she is well with no other health problems, a sensible target would be ≤ 6.5%. Diet alone is not achieving this target and control is likely to deteriorate with time.

The choice of OHA lies between metformin and a sulphonylurea. Whilst not overweight, she is likely to gain weight with a sulphonylurea. Metformin 500 mg twice daily is a reasonable choice, with low-dose sulphonylurea possible but carrying a risk of hypoglycaemia.

### CASE VIGNETTE 5.3

A frail 79-year-old lady was recently diagnosed following the death of her husband; she now lives alone. She is overweight (70 kg) with a BMI of 29 kg/m² on diet only. Her latest results are fasting glucose 8.3 mmol/l, HbA1c 7.5% and creatinine 118 μmol/l.

*Comment*

This seems similar to Cases 5.1 and 5.2 but the decision here is not clear-cut, either scientifically or clinically. Firstly, the relevant studies did not include patients in this age group. Secondly, the recommendation to control glucose levels tightly is on the basis of preventing long-term complications over 10–20 years. Realistically, she may not live long enough to reap the benefits.

However, in an otherwise healthy woman, it would be reasonable to treat, but – with her recent bereavement and living alone – waiting may be preferable. Additionally she is overweight with mild renal impairment that would make you hesitant to use metformin. In the elderly, glomerular filtration rate is significantly impaired even though serum creatinine is only minimally raised. Her calculated GFR is 39 ml/min (*see Box 14.2*).

A low-dose sulphonylurea such as gliclazide or glipizide could be considered (though she may not be eating well or regularly) but not glibenclamide because of the risk of prolonged hypoglycaemia while alone.

## THIAZOLIDINEDIONES – THE 'GLITAZONES'

### 5.13  What role is there for the 'glitazones' (thiazolidinediones, TZDs)?

These agents (rosiglitazone and pioglitazone) have recently been introduced and work on the PPAR-gamma receptor to reduce insulin resistance.[3,15] Unfortunately publication of data has been slow and outcome results are not yet available.[16] In general the TZDs produce similar glycaemic improvements (1.0–1.5%) to other agents, both as monotherapy and as combined therapy.

Currently TZDs are expensive and have no evidence of superiority though there are reasonably plausible claims (but little hard evidence) that they:

- maintain effect in the long term and preserve beta-cell function
- have beneficial effects on lipids and many other cardiovascular risk factors.

Current use is limited by licensing and funding issues, together with diminishing concerns about hepatic toxicity and their side effects, particularly weight gain, oedema and heart failure. The hepatotoxicity anxiety is probably unfounded, dating back to an earlier compound, troglitazone – indeed there is increasing evidence that TZDs may benefit fatty liver (*see Q. 18.2*). Clinical outcome trials are in progress but results are some years away.

Thiazolidinediones *take several months to show their full effect* so doses should not be rapidly adjusted and patients must be warned to be patient! Monitoring results is often helpful, but reviewing the HbA1c 3–6 months after starting a thiazolidinedione is the most valuable assessment. Trials with these drugs at full dosage suggest an approximate 1–1.5% reduction in HbA1c: if the patient is highly symptomatic or has an HbA1c >10%, it would usually be preferable to choose a faster-acting drug.

### 5.14  What are the side effects of the 'glitazones'?

Though it is now clear that rosiglitazone and pioglitazone carry no major risk of hepatic damage, manufacturers still advise performing 2-monthly liver function tests for the first year. The remaining common side effects are weight gain (a mean of 2–5 kg in most studies), together with oedema and haemodilution. There is concern about precipitation of heart failure, especially in patients on insulin, though it is somewhat unclear if the oedema is being used as a diagnostic marker for this. Glitazones should not at present be used in patients with heart failure or at very high risk for it. Their use with insulin should also be limited to specialists until more trial data are available.

## ACARBOSE

### 5.15 What role should acarbose play?

Acarbose is an inhibitor of alpha-glucosidase, thus limiting and delaying the absorption of starches. It has a mild hypoglycaemic effect, perhaps a mean HbA1c reduction of around 0.5% but at the expense of frequent gastrointestinal side effects including flatulence – these often cause patient withdrawal. It has a small role in patients unable to tolerate metformin and in combination therapy.

A recent study also showed a mild protective action in preventing conversion from impaired glucose tolerance (IGT) to diabetes.[10]

## PRACTICAL ASPECTS OF USING ORAL HYPOGLYCAEMIC AGENTS

### 5.16 How quickly can the dose of OHAs be adjusted?

This depends on the drug, as shown in *Figure 5.1*. Remember also that HbA1c will take 6–8 weeks to reach a plateau once control is stable. Self-tested or laboratory glucoses may be more useful, though fasting BGs alone can be misleading.

In practice drug doses are often not titrated up to maximal effect; it is often useful to make clear to the patient and in clinical notes what the next step should be if a goal is not achieved within a set period.

### 5.17 Which combinations of oral agents work best together?

Classically this has been metformin or sulphonylurea or the reverse! There are now more options, though good clinical trial data are limited[17,18] (*Table 5.4*). Triple therapy is currently being tested in trials and in the short term appears to be effective.[19] It is important to recognise that sometimes insulin is a better option and has proven benefit. (*See Case vignettes 5.4 and 5.5.*)

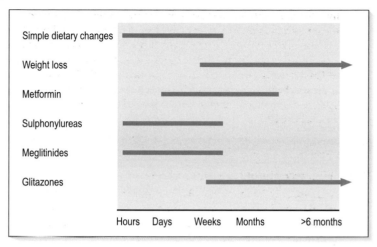

▲

**Fig. 5.1** Schematic of approximate onset of action and time to stability for various hypoglycaemic interventions.

## Table 5.4 Possible oral combination therapies[17-19]

| Drugs | Comments |
|---|---|
| Metformin first, then sulphonylurea | Most commonly used combination Some concerns about degree of benefit/safety |
| Sulphonylurea first, then metformin | Only likely to work if significant insulin resistance. Avoid if patient thin |
| Metformin plus TZD | Promising combination for insulin resistant/obese patients |
| Sulphonylurea plus TZD | Normally used when metformin not tolerated |
| 'Triple therapy' (metformin, SU + TZD) | Untested in long term. Insulin an alternative. Trials in progress |
| Metformin plus meglitinide | Limited data – should be effective |
| Metformin plus acarbose | Limited data |
| Sulphonylurea plus meglitinide | No real sense to combination |

SU, sulphonylurea; TZD, thiazolidinedione.

**CASE VIGNETTE 5.4**

A 48-year-old man has had type 2 diabetes for 3 years. BMI has fallen to 28.7 kg/m$^2$ while on treatment with metformin 850 mg twice daily. His fasting glucose is 8.5 mmol/l, HbA1c 7.8% and creatinine 94 µmol/l.

*Comment*

Glycaemic control here is not optimal, though not bad. For a patient on OHAs with no other serious illness, the target would usually be an HbA1c of 6.5–7.0%. The dose of metformin could be increased to 850 mg three times daily or 1 g twice daily assuming compliance. This may be insufficient to achieve optimal control, so the next step would be to add a sulphonylurea or a TZD.

**CASE VIGNETTE 5.5**

A very obese man (BMI 39 kg/m$^2$), aged 57 years, with type 2 diabetes and hypertension for 3 years is on maximal metformin 850 mg t.d.s. Results: fasting PG 9.1 mmol/l, HbA1c 8.4%, creatinine 105 µmol/l.

*Comment*

This is above any recommended target for HbA1c but this man is markedly overweight and, with his hypertension, he is likely to have the metabolic syndrome and significant insulin resistance.

Encouraging weight loss and exercise is obviously important but usually unsuccessful after 3 years. If he were keen to lose weight *and makes a good start with diet and exercise*, then addition of orlistat could be considered and has been shown to improve glycaemic control in type 2 diabetes provided there is weight reduction.

However, an additional OHA is likely to be required. It is more logical to combine a TZD with metformin than to add a sulphonylurea. This should lead to improved glycaemic control through increasing insulin sensitivity. His liver function tests should be checked before starting TZDs and regularly for the first year: it may take 2–4 months to see the effect of TZDs, a full dose probably being required to reach the desired target.

---

### 5.18 After starting an OHA, the patient has complained of hypoglycaemic episodes. As glycaemic control is still not good enough, what is the next step?

First obtain a clear history of the symptoms, to be sure they are hypoglycaemic in character, their frequency and the time of day they occur. If they are happening infrequently with a clear precipitating event (e.g. spring-cleaning the house), then reassurance and advice about prevention is adequate. If they are occurring frequently, then treatment needs adjustment. Hypoglycaemic episodes need to be avoided since they are unpleasant, and lead to additional food intake and weight gain. A reduced dose of OHA with no need to snack is better than a higher dose with extra eating, especially if the patient is obese. Some patients need to reduce or omit sulphonylureas before vigorous work/exercise – self-tested BGs are helpful here.

For some people with recently diagnosed type 2 diabetes, the fall in PG levels can lead to hypoglycaemic symptoms at levels of 4–6 mmol/l. Before diagnosis they have become habituated to much higher PG levels and an abrupt fall can produce 'hypoglycaemic' symptoms. This is the probable explanation for such symptoms in people treated with metformin alone since this does not cause true 'hypoglycaemia'. Reassurance and patience are required and, within a few weeks, the brain (which is the sensor for hypoglycaemia) becomes accustomed to the lower, normal, glucose levels.

The timing of tablet treatment can be adjusted to minimise hypoglycaemia. Medication is often given with breakfast, a relatively small meal, and many people are at their most active during the morning – thus hypoglycaemic symptoms mid- or late morning are common. It can be worth changing the timing of tablet treatment to later in the day with a main meal.

Finally, don't expect maximal improvement too soon (*see Q. 5.16*): HbA1c targets should be achieved 6 months after diagnosis but not necessarily at 3 months, especially if weight loss and increased exercise programmes are continuing.

## 5.19 How long should I persist with oral hypoglycaemic agents?

In general, for as long as they are well tolerated and achieving glycaemic goals. Clearly most people with type 2 diabetes will eventually progress to needing insulin, if they live long enough. The rate of progression varies widely but appears to be fairly consistent within an individual. Over the years there will tend to be a relentless, if slow, trend to a need for escalating therapy, as shown in *Figure 5.2*.

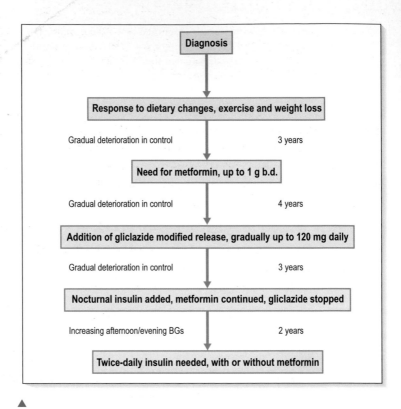

**Fig. 5.2** A typical example of the rate of progression in type 2 diabetes from diagnosis to the need for insulin. Note progression of treatment escalation varies widely between people with type 2 diabetes. (Note: gliclazide MR 120 mg daily is equivalent to gliclazide 160 mg b.d.)

# Insulin treatment

# 6

## TYPES OF INSULIN

### 6.1    How are the different types of insulin best classified?

The most practicable way is by their length of action (*Fig. 6.1*) rather than species of origin or means of manufacture, though the latter are important to some patients. A simple summary is given in *Table 6.1*, based on the UK but with some alternative drug names. The main manufacturers (Novo Nordisk, Eli Lilly and Aventis) are very helpful in providing details for travellers (*see Appendix 3*).

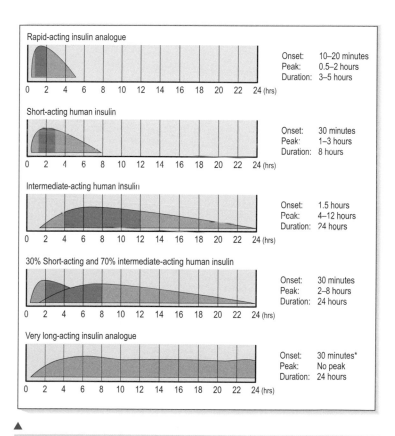

**Fig. 6.1** Approximate length of action of insulin preparations. The effective length of action also increases with increasing dose. *In repeated dosing, the 30 minute onset phase should disappear.

**TABLE 6.1 Guideline to insulin actions***

| Insulin type | Onset | Peak | Complete by |
|---|---|---|---|
| **Ultra-short acting insulins (analogues)** <br> Insulin aspart (NovoRapid) <br> Insulin lispro (Humalog) | 15–30 mins | 60–90 mins | 3–5 hours |
| **Short-acting insulins (soluble, neutral)** <br> Human soluble (Human Actrapid/Velosulin; <br> Humulin S/Humulin R; Insuman Rapid) | 30–60 mins | 120–240 mins | 6–8 hours |
| **Intermediate insulin (isophane)** <br> Human intermediate (Human <br> Insulatard/Protophane; Humulin I or N; <br> Insuman Basal) | 1–2 hours | 4–8 hours | 16–24 hours |
| **Longer-acting insulins (zinc-based)** <br> Human (Human Monotard; Humulin Lente; <br> Humulin Zn) | 1–3 hours | 4–12 hours | 16–24 hours |
| **Ultra-long acting insulin (analogue)** <br> Glargine (Lantus) | 2–4 hours | 4–24 hours | 24–36 hours |
| **Mixed insulins** | | Timings and proportions dependent upon preparation <br> Combinations of the above – ranges change from time to time | |
| Mixtard 10/Penmix 10 – Mixtard 50/Penmix 50 <br> Humulin M1/Humulin 90/10 – Humulin <br> M5/Humulin 50/50 <br> Insuman Com 15, 25, 50 | } from 10–50% soluble, 50–90% isophane | | |
| Novomix 30 <br> Humalog Mix 25/Mix 50 | } Combination of short analogues and isophane <br> Number indicates proportion of ultra-short insulin | | |

* This guideline to insulin actions is a rough estimate. Experience should make you aware that there is significant variability between patients. When large doses of insulin are injected, the duration of action increases significantly.

For non-human and less common insulins, consult the BNF or equivalent, or enquire from local insulin manufacturers.

## 6.2 What are the benefits of the new short-acting analogue insulins?

There are six main advantages of lispro- and aspart-insulins (Humalog and NovoRapid):[1]

- The insulin profiles more closely match blood glucose curves after meals.
- They can be given with food, not 20–30 minutes beforehand, which is more convenient and safer.
- They reduce the frequency of hypoglycaemia, especially before the next meal and in the early overnight period.
- In some patients, overall control is improved.
- They reduce the need for snacks between meals.
- They give flexibility in meals, both timing and quantity.

These analogues start working sooner (within 30 minutes), peak earlier (1–2 hours) and finish sooner, working for 3–4 hours, whereas short-acting 'soluble' insulins work for up to 6–8 hours. They are used at the time of eating (even slightly afterwards, for example in fussy children) and the insulin 'profile' more closely matches that of glucose from the absorbed food.

Humalog and NovoRapid have indistinguishable time profiles.

## 6.3 Are there any problems with the analogue insulins?

Because they only work for 3–4 hours, there is a risk of running out of insulin and patients therefore require a good basal insulin regimen. Clinical trials with these insulins with a single bedtime injection of intermediate-acting (isophane) insulin failed to show significant improvements in HbA1c despite the reduced frequency of hypos; when combined with twice-daily intermediate insulin, generally hypos were reduced and control improved. They also work well using insulin glargine[2,3] with its 24-hour duration.

Good patient understanding is fundamental to optimal use. Patients need to understand the concept that analogue insulins prevent the postprandial 'spikes' in blood glucose (BG), and need to be taken with food. Also, if taken too early, they can produce hypoglycaemia before food is absorbed, and if too big a dose is used, they produce hypoglycaemia after the meal. People need to experiment a little with doses, food and monitoring. There is a definite 'learning curve' when patients are switched to the analogues.

## 6.4 What are the advantages of glargine as a basal insulin?

Glargine has a very long half-life and produces nearly a 'plateau' in terms of its blood levels with a single daily dose.[4] For many patients this provides an easy basal insulin. Trials in type 1 and type 2 diabetes have shown that it is often equally effective given in the morning, at dinnertime or bedtime.[2] This should not vary from day to day: patients choose the most suitable time for their routine. Many patients have opted for a morning dose and feel a sense of freedom when no more injections are needed later in the day, though this does not work for all.

When insulin glargine was compared with isophane as the basal insulin in a multiple injection regimen, there was a significant reduction in night-time hypoglycaemic episodes.[3] Fasting BG levels were also better controlled. In initial trials HbA1c was not significantly improved but a more recent study[5] demonstrated a 0.4% reduction in well-controlled patients.

Apart from fewer hypos, a major advantage of using glargine is the ability to miss or significantly delay meals. On other regimens, the insulin may 'run out' and BG levels rise as the liver pours out glucose. The long duration of glargine means an effective control of liver gluconeogenesis. So, for patients who dislike eating breakfast or want to miss lunch occasionally, this is now possible. This has led to some successfully losing weight when transferred to glargine.

Another longer-acting insulin, detemir, will be available shortly. It is not as long lasting as glargine but may show less variability of absorption than any existing long-acting preparation. It may have a role especially as a nocturnal insulin and in combination with short-acting analogues. Interestingly, it appears to be associated with less weight gain than other insulins.

---

### 6.5    Are all insulins genetically engineered?

All the human and analogue insulins are made using some aspect of genetic engineering. This is done by placing a gene for the human insulin molecule inside a bacterium that is thus fooled into producing insulin. This insulin, which is of exactly the same genetic and chemical sequence as the normal 'self-made' human variety, is purified from the bacterial 'soup'. For those patients who have religious, ethical, 'green' or clinical problems with human insulins, there remains a selection of purified pork and beef insulins available in most countries (see the *BNF* or local pharmacopoeia, or ask manufacturers).

## WHEN TO USE INSULIN

### 6.6  What are the targets of treatment with insulin in type 2 diabetes?

These can be summarised as:
- *Patient well-being*, both freedom from symptoms of hyperglycaemia and positive wellness (e.g. improved energy).
- *Avoidance of hypoglycaemia*, either symptomatic or biochemical, and the anxiety surrounding it.
- *Optimal glycaemic control achievable for that individual patient.* Many authorities have extensively discussed this: most guidelines now recommend HbA1c values of ≤ 6.5–7.5% (*see Q. 2.12*) though there are dissenting voices, suggesting this is unachievable for many patients, especially the elderly and frail for whom the dangers outweigh the benefits.[6]

In type 2 diabetes, there is little evidence to support the proposed targets for patients' self-testing BG levels. However, those outlined in *Table 6.2* are based on day-to-day practice, the lowest range being chosen for patients in whom optimal glycaemic control is absolutely vital (e.g. the younger type 2 patient with complications), the middle range for patients in whom hypoglycaemia needs to be minimised while maintaining good control (e.g. a driver), with the highest range being more suited for those elderly, frail or high-risk individuals in whom avoidance of hypoglycaemia and simple freedom from hyperglycaemic symptoms are most important.

Targets for glycaemic control need to be agreed with each individual patient and not simply imposed – otherwise there will be little motivation to achieve them. There has been limited research on what patients perceive as worthwhile risk reductions.[7] The long-term benefit of fewer diabetic complications needs to be balanced carefully by the patient against an increased risk of hypoglycaemia (*see Q. 7.7*). Also, all the usual factors influencing choice of therapy (e.g. exercise/sport, driving, dexterity, memory) will have an impact on the patient's final decision.

### TABLE 6.2  Target ranges for self-testing of blood glucose levels

| Type of patient | Fasting and pre-prandial (mmol/l) | Post-prandial (mmol/) |
| --- | --- | --- |
| Optimal control essential | 4–5.5 | 4–8 |
| The majority | 4–7 | 4–10 |
| High hypoglycaemia risk | 5–8 | 5–11 |

## 6.7 When should insulin be introduced in type 2 diabetes?

There is no simple answer. Better understanding of the pathophysiology of type 2 diabetes with progressive loss of beta-cell function and thus insulin secretion has driven a re-evaluation of insulin usage (*Fig. 6.2*). Previously, it was used as a last resort, often started only when patients were symptomatic from uncontrolled hyperglycaemia. Recognising that most patients with type 2 diabetes will eventually need insulin 'replacement' has produced a re-evaluation of the approach to patient management and education – many physicians now discuss this with patients soon after diagnosis, though individuals vary in the degree of beta-cell damage at diagnosis and the subsequent rate of insulin secretory loss. It is important that optimal treatment is seen as the target and insulin use as a natural progression in therapy.

Previously, most patients taking a combination of the maximum dose of oral hypoglycaemic agents (OHAs) would reach an HbA1c of 9–11% before insulin was started. Now, national and international targets encourage HbA1c levels of around or below 7%, and insulin is increasingly being started in patients who are asymptomatic in relation to hyperglycaemia. Nowadays, for many patients, insulin conversion will occur when HbA1c is

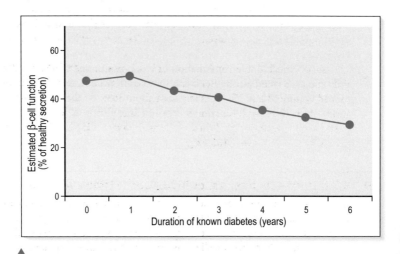

**Fig. 6.2** Progressive loss of beta-cell function with time in type 2 diabetes. Note that approximately 50% of secretory capacity is already lost at the time of diagnosis.

around 8% and there is still some residual insulin secretion. Full 'replacement' therapy (as in type 1 diabetes with both short- and long-acting insulins) is usually unnecessary. This has led to the development of 'nocturnal' insulin therapy, with one dose of intermediate- or long-acting insulin given at bedtime, while continuing with daytime OHAs.

However, past experience with patients in the Poole Department of Diabetes found little improvement in control in patients converted to insulin when HbA1c was initially 8–9%. This was using a twice-daily pre-mixed regimen and recent use of night-time insulin with OHAs is more promising.

## 6.8 When is combination therapy, with insulin and an oral agent, indicated?

Several studies, mainly from Scandinavia, have shown this to be an effective treatment when there is significant beta-cell failure but still some residual secretion.[8] The usual regimen has a nocturnal isophane insulin (e.g. Insulatard, also known as Protophane) with daytime metformin or a sulphonylurea. The insulin works largely by suppressing hepatic gluconeogenesis overnight but tends to lead to BG 'escape' in the late afternoon. The combination with metformin leads to less weight gain, better glycaemic control and an improved lipid profile.[9]

Increasingly in the UK, the long-acting insulin, glargine, is being introduced in patients taking both a sulphonylurea and metformin.[10] Stopping one of these OHAs when commencing insulin leads to higher doses of insulin being required and a longer time to stabilisation of glucose levels.

As a practical hint, a combination of basal insulin and OHAs usually only succeeds when fasting BG is less than 10–11 mmol/l, few daytime values exceed 15 mmol/l and HbA1c is less than about 10%. As the years pass, further loss of beta-cell function means daytime glucose levels rise, particularly after meals, and then additional doses of daytime insulin are necessary (*see Q. 6.9 and Table 6.3*).

## 6.9 What insulin regimens should be used in type 2 diabetes?

Earlier use of insulin means there is often substantial residual endogenous insulin secretion, which permits use of nocturnal insulins to suppress hepatic glucose production overnight and controlling fasting BG levels (*see Q. 6.4*). Comparative studies have shown that continuing daytime metformin minimises weight gain, which is a particularly suitable regimen for the great majority of patients with type 2 diabetes who are overweight (*see Q. 6.8*).

Choice of insulin regimens beyond the straightforward is a skilled task with little hard evidence. For non-experts, familiarity with a few is more appropriate than occasional use of many. Lifestyle factors and patient preference often drive the final choice: specialist advice is wise when there are difficulties, for example with poor control, hypoglycaemia or difficulty in adherence.

*Table 6.3* shows some of the commoner regimens, together with their advantages and disadvantages.

---

### 6.10 What are the differences in treatment regimens for type 1 diabetes?

After 2–5 years of type 1 diabetes there is usually little or no residual insulin secretion. Thus the administered insulin regimen attempts to mimic physiological replacement, which has a basal insulin component with rapid post-prandial (and post-snack) surges in insulin to control the post-prandial glucose rise (*see Q. 6.3*). Such regimens almost always require some short-acting insulin, whereas those in type 2 diabetes sometimes do not while there is still significant residual insulin secretion.

The commonly used insulin regimens are shown as numbers 6–9 in *Table 6.3*, though many more have been advocated, often without appropriate comparative studies. The list includes the most common usage in European-based countries (including Australia, New Zealand and South Africa), though availability and nomenclature differ between countries.

Multiple injection regimens, involving 3–5 injections per day (most often 4), are widely used though they do require good education of a co-operative patient; they, together with pumps, have been the basis of intensive treatment trials such as the DCCT.[11]

Where someone is not well controlled on one of these regimens, specialist advice should be sought, as there are many causes of poor control, often reflecting issues beyond choice of an appropriate insulin regimen.

**TABLE 6.3  Insulin regimens in type 2 diabetes**

| Insulin regimen | Advantages | Problems | Best suited for |
|---|---|---|---|
| 1 Bedtime intermediate + metformin | Simple<br>Convenient<br>Least weight gain<br>Benefits on cardiovascular risk | Higher BGs in p.m./evening | Patients with early beta-cell failure; overweight or obese (i.e. most!) |
| 2 Bedtime intermediate + sulphonylureas/other secretagogues | Simple<br>Convenient | Higher BGs in p.m./evening<br>Weight gain | Patients with early beta-cell failure; slim or normal weight |
| 3 Once-daily glargine | Simple<br>Convenient<br>Very long acting | Limited evidence yet<br>Possible unpredictability | Patients with early beta-cell failure |
| 4 Once-daily glargine + metformin/sulphonylurea | Simple | Limited evidence as yet | Patients with early beta-cell failure |
| 5 Twice-daily intermediate | Relatively simple | Poor control of post-prandial BGs | ?Next stage in the obese, but check post-prandial BGs |
| 6 Twice-daily pre-mixed insulin | Relatively simple | Weight gain<br>Hypoglycaemia risk | Often a compromise when more complex regimens unacceptable |
| 7 Twice-daily custom mixed mixed short- and long-acting insulins | Flexible | Needs skill/judgement<br>Hypoglycaemia risk | Patients wanting flexibility to adjust short- and long-acting doses separately but who wish to stay on twice daily insulin; they have usually tried pre-mixed and had problems |
| 8 Three times daily: a.m. intermediate + sulphonylurea; p.m, sulphonylurea; bedtime intermediate | Flexible | Quite complex<br>Hypoglycaemia | Younger able patients; often good if nocturnal hypos an issue. Use short-acting sulphonylureas or meglitinide |
| 9 Multi-injection regimens | Very flexible | Complex | Younger intelligent patients |

## HOW TO START INSULIN IN PRACTICE

### 6.11 How should the transfer to insulin be managed?

This is best summarised in several steps:
1. Discussing the need with the patient, preferably well beforehand (*see Q. 6.7*).
2. Educating the individual, and possibly the family or carers.
3. Starting the insulin.
4. Titrating the insulin dose, and achieving agreed targets.
5. Changing/phasing out some or all OHAs.
   Patients easily lose confidence at this time, so this is not something to be undertaken occasionally. An experienced diabetes nurse is usually the best person to manage the change, and to shepherd the patient through this often anxious period (*see also Case vignettes 5.4, 5.5 and 8.1–8.3*).

### 6.12 What does a patient need to know about starting insulin?

There are a number of areas to cover:
- How, where and when to inject a given dose – 'pen' or syringe
- Possible changes in diet and/or exercise patterns
- Prevention, detection and treatment of hypoglycaemia
- Appropriate blood testing
- Dose titration and adjustment
- What to do in the event of illness.

### 6.13 What should be the starting dose of insulin?

A difficult question to answer – there is no 'right' dose for all patients with type 2 diabetes. Insulin should only be commenced by a health care professional with experience: there are no proven algorithms for initial or final doses, and even experienced diabetologists sometimes get this wrong.

Some basic guidance can be given:

- Start with a low dose, then gradually increase according to self-tested BG levels over several days. This reduces the risk of hypoglycaemia.
- The more obese the patient, the more likely eventual doses will be high.
- Initial high BG levels do not always imply eventual high doses.
- Encourage patients to be involved in their own dose changes, and ultimately to take over dose titration using the targets shown in *Table 6.2*.

*Nocturnal insulin*

With nocturnal insulin, start with 0.1–0.2 units/kg (often 8–16 units for obese patients with type 2 diabetes) and increase gradually every 4–7 days using the fasting BG as the guide. Most would continue OHAs until fasting BG levels are below 10 mmol/l before stopping the least necessary OHA (e.g. sulphonylurea in overweight patients, metformin in the thin) if this is the planned eventual treatment. Average doses of nocturnal insulin are 30–40 units when combined with metformin; many authorities do not exceed 0.5 units/kg as a single nocturnal dose, preferring then to use twice-daily insulin, large single doses contributing to hypoglycaemia.

*Twice-daily insulin*

Start with around 0.2 units/kg (e.g. 6–10 units before breakfast and dinner), usually split with around 60% in the morning, 40% in the evening unless there are good reasons to do otherwise (e.g. heavy physical daytime work). While metformin may be continued in the overweight, sulphonylureas and other secretagogues are usually withdrawn. Insulin requirements often reach 0.7–1.5 units/kg/day, or more.

 Insulin leads to weight gain, less so when combined with metformin, but sometimes a vicious circle develops with increasing amounts of insulin needed to control BG levels while weight and insulin resistance increase. Patients frequently feel hungry on insulin, aggravating the problem. Once insulin doses have reached 1 unit/kg, it is worth reviewing whether increasing the insulin doses in the last few weeks has led to any improvement in control. Further increases may just fuel further insulin resistance. It is reasonable to wait a few weeks at this dose of insulin as one frequently sees BG levels fall during this time. The mechanism of this is unclear but it may relate to some improvement in endogenous beta-cell function.

The role of thiazolidinediones in this situation is still unclear, and their use is only recommended under specialist supervision: this indication is not licensed in many countries (*see also Case vignettes 5.4, 5.5 and 8.1–8.3*).

---

### 6.14 Can patients adjust their own insulin doses in type 2 diabetes?

Yes, this should be the goal for most patients. Effective education will encourage the patient or carer to undertake subsequent adjustment, especially where lifestyle is variable from day to day or week to week. The principles need to be carefully taught by an experienced health care professional: this role is generally undertaken by the diabetes nurse specialist who will then continue to support the patient as they learn through day-to-day experience.

Important educational pointers include:

■ length of action of the insulin preparation, when it peaks and wears off
■ the timing of injections, and how they relate to meals and snacks
■ the pattern of exercise, whether at work or as sport/hobbies
■ the influence of injection sites and technique
■ the natural variability of insulin absorption following subcutaneous injections
■ the use of the fasting BG as the best guide to evening/bedtime insulin dose.

In general, patients are advised to adjust insulin doses by 2–4 units at a time and wait for at least 3 days to see the effect of the change. With experience, some will adjust doses in relation to food intake and varying activity on a much more frequent basis. Patients need to be encouraged that they can and should adjust doses if control according to their own monitoring results is not ideal.

## PROBLEMS AND ISSUES IN USING INSULIN

### 6.15 What about patients with needle phobia?

With careful preparation and education, this is actually rare. Many diabetes units now make clear to all patients with type 2 diabetes that insulin will probably be needed eventually. Demonstrating an injection often overcomes many of the fears and people can even try themselves (with saline!) before they need insulin.

A few people do have genuine phobias and may need formal psychological help, but many others can be persuaded in time to give insulin a trial for 12 weeks with a return to tablets if no benefit is gained. Very few choose to revert. The recent introduction of the needleless injector device can be helpful in some difficult cases. The device works by high pressure forcing the insulin into the subcutaneous tissue. It is not clear whether these devices will lead to significant problems with lipohypertrophy or atrophy which can affect insulin absorption and action.

### 6.16 Don't many patients prove very resistant to insulin?

Yes – if only we knew the answer to this one! Many obese patients simply put on weight when started on insulin (at least 2–4 kg) and need an ever-increasing dose to try to achieve control, which puts on more weight; they then become more insulin resistant so need yet more … and so on. This has been described as the 'insulin sink' syndrome. One small and incomplete solution is to continue metformin, which reduces the degree of weight gain and insulin need (perhaps 10–20% less insulin).[8,12] Trials are taking place of the 'glitazones' as an obvious solution, but these drugs tend to increase weight anyway.

In practice, a decision has to be made as to which compromise of control and weight is best for the individual patient – an optimal solution is rarely present with current tools.

### 6.17 Doesn't human insulin cause severe unrecognised hypoglycaemia?

This was an enormous concern when 'human' insulin was first introduced. Multiple trials have shown no systemic difference between human and animal insulins in hypoglycaemic responses though it is entirely possible that, for a few individuals, this is so.[13] Animal insulins are therefore still available.

In retrospect it is likely that many of the reports associated with the introduction of human insulin related to the period of intensifying glycaemic control in the 1980s. Until that time the frequency and importance of hypoglycaemia and hypoglycaemic unawareness had not been adequately recognised.

### 6.18 Why does the dose vary so much between patients?

There is no satisfactory explanation for the wide range of doses needed in type 1 diabetes, though worldwide the *average* is remarkably constant at about 0.7 units/kg/day for adults. It is much higher during adolescence at around 1.1–1.2 units/kg/day. However, there are many patients controlled for years on 10–20 units/day whereas others need over 100 units/day.

Similar variability is seen in type 2 diabetes. Obesity and presumed insulin resistance would make one expect a high dose, but some people are well controlled on 10–20 units daily. Higher doses are rather commoner in type 2 diabetes with many patients needing 1–2 units/kg/day – insulin resistance is usually defined as >2 units/kg/day.

### 6.19 What causes the instability I see in many of my insulin-treated patients?

This is common and has several components, any or all of which may be relevant for an individual:

- Subcutaneous injection of insulin produces highly variable blood insulin levels on different days, even with optimal injection technique.
- Injection site problems (lipohypertrophy and atrophy) are common and amplify the variability.
- Subcutaneous insulin is not a truly physiological replacement – the pancreas secretes insulin into the portal circulation (*see Q. 1.2*).
- Patient habits, meals and exercise often vary widely.
- Stress substantially affects the pattern for many people.

### 6.20 What about insulin pumps?

Insulin pumps as a delivery method are widely used for patients with type 1 diabetes in the US but are expensive to buy and run. They additionally require substantial educational and medical input and a well-motivated patient.[14] In other countries, they are usually reserved for individuals with particular problems:

■ 'brittle' diabetes – frequent alternating hyperglycaemia/diabetic ketoacidosis and hypoglycaemia (official definitions usually include multiple admissions)
■ hypoglycaemia unawareness
■ patients with unpredictable lifestyles (e.g. shift workers)
■ situations where optimal glycaemic control is mandatory (e.g. pregnancy).

These are a specialist area, even within diabetes units.

### 6.21 Are there any other issues with insulin?

Other problems include:

■ *Injection site hypertrophy*: Recurrent injection into the same site causes lipohypertrophy – this makes insulin absorption more variable. It is a common issue, and examination of sites should be part of the annual review – you cannot always believe the patient who assures you they rotate their sites!
■ *Insulin allergy*: This is now very rare. When seen, it is usually due to a stabiliser used in insulin preparations. In older patients using old (impure) animal insulins it was more common, then being due to non-insulin proteins.
■ *Insulin oedema*: This unusual phenomenon is occasionally seen after a newly diagnosed or very poorly controlled patient is started/restarted on insulin. Mild to moderate nondescript ankle oedema develops over a few days to weeks, and then spontaneously goes, again over a few weeks. Anecdotally it is commonest in young women with type 1 diabetes using insulin omission as a weight loss technique.

### 6.22 Are there alternative delivery methods available for insulin?

Delivering insulin by inhaler has been shown to work, mimicking a rapid-acting insulin analogue in its absorption. Full clinical trials are underway to establish safety and reliability in long-term use. Other potential methods include oral formulations and transdermal delivery but these are less advanced.

# PQ PATIENT QUESTIONS

## 6.23 But a friend of a friend died soon after they were started on insulin.

This is a common (and often unspoken) fear that usually goes back to the days when insulin was used as a last resort. Such patients were put onto insulin in the last days, weeks or months of their life, usually already suffering from multiple problems (usually kidney and cardiac) from their diabetes. It would have been these problems that caused their death, not the late change to insulin.

We now know that good control substantially reduces the chance of these complications, and doctors and patients are using insulin much earlier to prevent the problems.

## 6.24 Can I change my own insulin dose?

Yes. This is encouraged and requires only simple knowledge, especially with overnight insulin. You need to understand:

- which insulin works when and for how long
- what affects your insulin needs – food, exercise, time of day
- which of your test results are most helpful.

(*See also Figure 6.1 and the answer to Question 6.14.*)

# Hypoglycaemia

# 7

## DEFINITION AND EPIDEMIOLOGY

### 7.1    What is the definition of hypoglycaemia?

This needs two answers, numerical and practical. In healthy individuals and most people with type 2 diabetes, hypoglycaemic symptoms (e.g. shakiness, sweating, difficulty in concentrating) would be detected at plasma glucose (PG) levels between 3.5 and 4 mmol/l and symptoms would increase as PG falls further. This range is significantly higher than the level at which spontaneous hypoglycaemia in a non-diabetic person is diagnosed (below 2.2 mmol/l), and also lower than that sometimes seen 3–5 hours after a glucose load and labelled 'reactive hypoglycaemia'.

'Severe' hypoglycaemia refers to an episode where the individual needs third-party assistance (from partner, friend or paramedic) to recover. 'Mild' hypoglycaemia refers to episodes self-diagnosed and self-treated without the need for external help. Pure 'biochemical' hypoglycaemia refers to recorded PG levels below a threshold, which varies between different research studies. Thus care is needed in interpreting studies where there may be different definitions of hypoglycaemia or methods of blood glucose (BG) measurement.

Most specialists encourage patients to avoid BG levels below 4 mmol/l, though this is often difficult to achieve in insulin-treated people. It is important to recognise that under most circumstances *capillary BG* (measured by meters) is about 0.2–0.5 mmol/l higher than *venous PG* (measured by laboratory techniques), the difference depending on absolute concentration of glucose and sluggishness of capillary circulation. Thus, a capillary BG of 4.0 probably represents a PG of about 3.5–3.8 mmol/l.

### 7.2    How common is hypoglycaemia in type 2 diabetes?

Fortunately, hypoglycaemia in type 2 diabetes is less common than in type 1 diabetes. However, it is still a major cause of emergency hospital admission, significant symptoms and real anxiety often limiting a patient's acceptance or adherence to therapy. Additionally, a number of patients have occupational limitations because of hypoglycaemia (see Ch. 11), particularly drivers of heavy goods and passenger service vehicles.

The best estimates would place the frequency of hypoglycaemia in type 2 diabetic patients on insulin at around 5–10% of that for type 1 diabetes; figures from recent trials in type 1 and type 2 diabetes are given in *Table 7.1*.[1–3]

Patients treated with sulphonylureas, and to a lesser extent with meglitinides,[4] have a lower, though still significant frequency of hypoglycaemia, especially in high-risk patients such as the elderly and those with impaired renal function. Severe hypoglycaemia caused by

**TABLE 7.1  Frequency of hypoglycaemia in major trials**

| Trial | Type of diabetes and treatment | Frequency |
|---|---|---|
| UKPDS[1] | Type 2 diabetes Intensive insulin treatment | One or more major hypoglycaemic episodes occurred in 2.3% of patients per year Any hypoglycaemic episode occurred in 36.5% of patients per year |
| Kumamoto[2] | Type 2 diabetes Intensive insulin treatment | No episodes of severe hypoglycaemia Mild hypo symptoms in 6 patients on intensive insulin therapy compared to 4 patients on conventional therapy |
| DCCT[3] | Type 1 diabetes Intensive insulin treatment | Severe hypoglycaemic episodes: 0.6 episodes per patient per year in intensive group compared to 0.2 in controls |

sulphonylurea therapy is an extremely dangerous condition and causes substantial morbidity and mortality.

All patients treated with hypoglycaemic therapy should be questioned about symptomatic or asymptomatic hypoglycaemia, and educated about how to recognise, avoid and treat it. As HbA1c 'targets' are reduced, the frequency of hypoglycaemia is intrinsically likely to increase.

## AWARENESS AND UNAWARENESS

### 7.3  How do people normally recognise and respond to hypoglycaemia?

In the healthy individual, endogenous pancreatic insulin secretion will cease when PG reaches around 4.5 mmol/l. Glucose is released from the liver glycogen stores when the inhibitory effect of insulin is withdrawn so PG will then rise. The diabetic individual on insulin or sulphonylurea treatment cannot 'switch off' insulin secretion, therefore PG may continue to fall. At glucose levels of 3.5–3.9 mmol/l, the brain normally institutes counter-regulatory measures involving activation of the sympathetic nervous system with a neuroendocrine release of catecholamines, glucagon, cortisol and growth hormone, all of which increase PG.[5–7]

Under normal circumstances, hypoglycaemia will be reversed by the mechanism shown in *Figure 7.1*. The neuroendocrine response also produces significant symptoms, warning the patient that PG is low and hopefully producing an intelligent response to take glucose-containing foods.

If PG continues to fall and the patient is unable to recognise the symptoms, the response mechanism is impaired and/or no food is eaten, the PG will continue to fall, eventually leading to impaired cognitive function and then to a 'neuroglycopenic' state with impairment of consciousness. This occurs at a lower level, normally below 2 mmol/l.

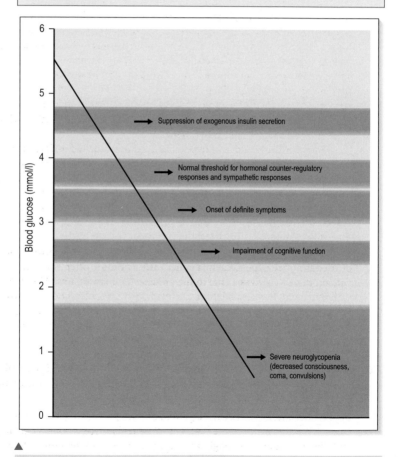

**Fig. 7.1** The progressive physiological response to increasing hypoglycaemia in a healthy individual.

### 7.4    Are there any rare manifestations of hypoglycaemia?

Rare presentations of hypoglycaemia include unusual behaviour, fits (often nocturnal) and fractures from fitting. Claiming that hypoglycaemia causes criminal behaviour is a recognised defence strategy in court, though used with variable success!

### 7.5    What is hypoglycaemic unawareness?

Repeated exposure to hypoglycaemia reduces the counter-regulatory responses and the PG threshold for autonomic/sympathetic activation may fall below the usual 3.5–3.9 mmol/l.[8] This appears to be an adaptive response, but the neuroglycopenic threshold does not alter significantly. The result is that the sympathetic responses may not occur until the threshold for neuroglycopenia has already been reached. The patient then only experiences the sympathetic warning symptoms when the brain is already neuroglycopenic and not functioning properly, so they are not recognised. At this stage, the patient may appear to go rapidly from apparent normality to impaired consciousness.[9,10] This is obviously potentially dangerous, especially for those whose work or normal activities involve machinery or high-risk situations.

With careful avoidance of hypoglycaemia, it is usually possible to re-establish the normal threshold for sympathetic symptoms again. However, this is often difficult to achieve in long-standing type 1 diabetes where there may be significant impairment of autonomic and endocrine responses. Rigorous hypoglycaemia avoidance is difficult, and recurrent hypoglycaemia or lack of awareness in anyone with diabetes is a strong indication for specialist referral.

In evaluating awareness, it is useful to ask if the patient's partner, family or friends notice hypoglycaemia either earlier or more often than the patient; this often gives a clue to the presence of unawareness. Also, any patient with an incidental laboratory PG below 4 mmol/l should be closely questioned about awareness of hypoglycaemia at that time. Many patients forget or fail to report hypoglycaemic episodes so detailed questioning of patient and family is vital. (*See also Case vignette 7.1.*)

### 7.6    My patient with type 2 diabetes claims to feel hypoglycaemic whenever his blood glucose is below 6 mmol/l. Is this possible?

Yes, this has been shown in patients who have previously been hyperglycaemic, either newly diagnosed or after periods of poor glycaemic control.[11] In this instance the reverse to the previous scenario is happening, with the threshold for hypoglycaemia rising as the brain habituates to high PG levels. Sudden improvement in control, most usually with intensive treatment, can then produce significant hypoglycaemic symptoms while PG is still in the 'normal range' of 4–7 mmol/l. Fortunately, gradual improvement in control will normally restore awareness to the usual thresholds described above. This is probably the mechanism for the occasional description of hypoglycaemia in patients treated with metformin alone, which should not be able to cause hypoglycaemia on its own.

## RISK FACTORS FOR HYPOGLYCAEMIA

### 7.7 Which patients with type 2 diabetes are at risk of hypoglycaemia?

 Biochemical hypoglycaemia (PG below 3.5 mmol/l) does not occur with diet/exercise alone or with metformin or 'glitazones' unless there is prolonged fasting.

Significant clinical hypoglycaemia therefore only occurs with insulin, sulphonylurea or meglitinide treatment. In type 2 diabetes, this is commonest in patients with very 'tight' control, those on multiple daily insulin injections and those on long-acting sulphonylureas, especially glibenclamide.

No consultation with a patient on insulin or sulphonylureas is complete without an enquiry about possible hypoglycaemia, clinical and biochemical. Physicians have often been lax about detecting and preventing what is one of our patients' greatest fears. People's understanding about hypoglycaemia varies considerably: many associate severe hypoglycaemia with loss of consciousness. Asking how often they have to eat extra because they feel their sugar may be low often reveals a surprising answer when problems with hypos have been denied.

### 7.8 What about risk factors for hypoglycaemia in type 1 diabetes?

 These are complex. Most studies have shown associations of hypoglycaemia with:
- previous hypoglycaemic episodes
- tight/intensive control regimens
- patients achieving HbA1c < 7%
- the presence of hypoglycaemic unawareness
- long duration of diabetes.

### 7.9 What are the main causes of hypoglycaemia?

These are usually one or more of: too much insulin or hypoglycaemic agent (e.g. sulphonylurea), too little food, delay/omission of a meal and increased exercise.

Hypoglycaemia is often the result of a combination of several factors, and careful history taking will usually elucidate the problem. Particular issues include:

- *Too much treatment*: the dose of insulin or oral hypoglycaemic agent (OHA)
- *Food*: frequently being late for or missing a meal, a small rushed meal or too little carbohydrate
- *Exercise*: this increases basal metabolic rate, often causing delayed hypoglycaemia many hours later
- *Inappropriate timing* of insulin or tablet taking
- *Injection site problems* such as intramuscular injection giving unusual absorption of insulin.

Hypoglycaemia on insulin is predictably most common before lunch, then before dinner, and then overnight (especially between 0300 and 0700 hours). A lie-in with a delayed breakfast will often cause it, especially after a day's exercise. Similar times are high risk with oral agents, though this will vary depending upon the agent used and its peak/duration of action together with dosing and meal timing. Long-acting sulphonylureas (e.g. glibenclamide) may often cause overnight hypoglycaemia.

Patients performing BG measurements should be encouraged to test at times of high risk for hypoglycaemia, or in the event of possible symptoms.

### 7.10 What are the less common causes of hypoglycaemia?

If hypoglycaemia is not easily dealt with, then referral is indicated. It should be urgent if there are frequent episodes or there is unawareness. Rarely there are other pathophysiological contributors such as hypothyroidism, hypopituitarism or Addison's disease, or other circumstances such as:

- hypoglycaemia in type 1 diabetes in early pregnancy, when insulin requirements may fall in the first trimester before they rise later (*see Ch. 12*)
- renal impairment leading to delayed excretion with prolongation and potentiation of insulin or sulphonylurea action
- syringe, insulin pen or pump malfunction (though more often patient error).

### 7.11 How important is exercise in causing hypoglycaemia?

The effect of exercise in increasing glucose disposal for many hours after its completion is often underestimated. Few people with diabetes become hypoglycaemic while on a normal walk or playing a standard sport of 1–2 hours, the common exceptions being 18 holes of golf, a long swimming/water sports session, ski-ing or an endurance sport. The metabolic rate and glucose disposal is increased for over 12 hours after vigorous exercise, so the hypoglycaemia may not immediately be related to the exercise. In many patients, it is necessary to decrease the dose of insulin or OHA before, and possibly after, strenuous activity is taken. This can often be seen if careful records are kept documenting BGs and exercise levels; strategies can then be devised to avoid hypoglycaemia. With obese patients it is more appropriate to decrease doses of insulin or OHAs than to take additional snacks or food (*see also Qs 4.18 and 4.19*).

One of the authors has a well-controlled golfing surgeon on low-dose gliclazide who tended to go hypoglycaemic on the 11th green, rarely earlier or later. The problem was solved by omitting the morning gliclazide on days when he was playing 18 holes; a round of 9 holes did not produce the same effect as he reached the 19th hole sooner!

Exercise problems often arise on unusually active holidays and weekends.

### 7.12 What are the differences in patients with type 1 diabetes?

Hypoglycaemia in type 1 diabetes is much commoner than in type 2 diabetes and is the major limitation to good control. Data from the DCCT showed an exponential rise in hypoglycaemia as mean HbA1c fell, thus a reduced risk of complications was balanced by an increased frequency of hypoglycaemia[3] (*Fig. 7.2*). This has been found in other studies, though more recent clinical trials involving the ultra-short-acting analogue insulins (Humalog and NovoRapid), combined in appropriate regimens, have shown a significant ($\approx$ 30%) reduction in the absolute rate of hypoglycaemia, especially for the late morning and overnight periods.

Similarly, the new long-acting basal insulin glargine has been shown to reduce overnight hypoglycaemic episodes in several studies. Better understanding of hypoglycaemia and newer insulins in the well-educated patient should lead to fewer hypoglycaemic problems than those seen in the DCCT (*see Q. 2.4*).

## CONSEQUENCES OF HYPOGLYCAEMIA

### 7.13 Isn't hypoglycaemia dangerous to the brain?

In severe instances, prolonged hypoglycaemia can cause death or serious brain injury. Fortunately this is far less common with insulin than people

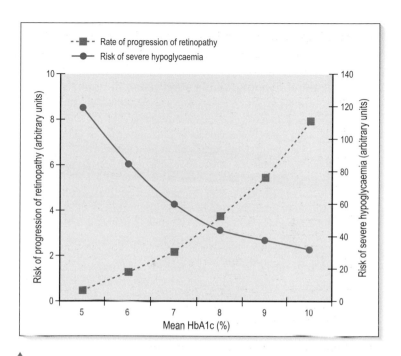

**Fig. 7.2** The relationship between glycaemic control, retinopathy risk and hypoglycaemia frequency in DCCT. (From DCCT Research Group[3] with permission from New England Journal of Medicine.)

commonly think. The body's counter-regulation mechanism will eventually respond, even if at a lower PG than normal. This results in recovery through the catecholamine, cortisol, glucagon and growth hormone effects, which include direct and/or indirect action to increase PG.

The exception is with sulphonylurea treatment when any rise in PG is promptly counterbalanced by further insulin secretion and recurrent hypoglycaemia that may persist or recur *for over 24 hours*, especially in the elderly or those with renal failure. The longer-acting agents (glibenclamide and chlorpropamide) are most dangerous and most authorities strongly recommend against their use in those at high risk: the elderly, the frail, those living alone and those with impaired renal function.

The effect of milder recurrent hypoglycaemia is still controversial. There is some, but far from conclusive, evidence in type 1 diabetes that recurrent hypoglycaemia in children may reduce intellectual performance both now and in later life. There is also the very rare 'dead-in-bed' syndrome that is thought, but not proven, to have a partly hypoglycaemic origin.

---

### 7.14 What about hypoglycaemia and driving in type 2 diabetes?

This controversial subject has been well reviewed by MacLeod.[12] There are few good data on the actual risks but available evidence does not suggest any substantial effect on accidents or mortality, though there are clearly a number of individual cases, nearly all in private car drivers.

Hypoglycaemia is not an issue for patients on lifestyle management alone or metformin by itself as their PG level will never fall into the range liable to cause neuroglycopenia. However, all patients on sulphonylureas, meglitinides or insulin should be taught about the risk of hypoglycaemia while driving and how to prevent and treat it. For these patients, private car licences are normally issued but heavy goods vehicle and passenger service licences may not be.

The issue should be of risk and hazard, but European Community (EC) regulations are currently rule- rather than risk-based. The *risk* of a hypoglycaemic episode while driving depends on:

- treatment type
- time exposed – the more hours driving, the higher the risk
- regularity of meals/snacks
- adherence to testing.

The *hazard*, if an accident should occur, relates to the potential damage caused by the vehicle, number of passengers/other road users, any danger of the cargo and the road conditions/crowding.

The risk is obviously greater in patients on insulin, though less in patients on nocturnal insulin/daytime OHA regimens than in those on multiple mixed insulins. In general, type 1 patients may not hold higher classes of licence, nor type 2 patients if treated with insulin.

Some countries such as New Zealand have more risk-based regimens, where individual rather than blanket decisions are made – and driving may be allowed under a number of strict conditions. The patient organisation Diabetes UK is currently promoting a similar approach in the UK; for recent news see the DVLA website (*www.dvla.gov.uk*). All such applications require a specialist report, so early referral is recommended as extended periods of observation and documentation may be needed.

All patients who drive should be advised about hypoglycaemia avoidance and treatment, ideally in a written form. A good description of the instructions is available on *www.ltsa.govt.nz*.

Driving is also considered in *Chapter 11*, and *see also Case vignette 7.1*.

### 7.15  How is this different for type 1 diabetes?

The risk is much higher in type 1 than in type 2 diabetes and most legal jurisdictions agree on substantial restrictions on driving passenger and heavy goods vehicles. In the UK, there is a small and diminishing number of drivers with type 1 diabetes who already hold these special licences. They have 'grandfather' rights but the DVLA requires an annual specialist examination and report (*see also www.ltsa.govt.nz*).

The clearest issue is hypoglycaemia unawareness, which is commoner in this group and is a complete bar to driving. Unawareness may be reversible with strict hypoglycaemia avoidance, which requires extensive specialist input (*see Q. 7.5 and Case vignette 7.1*).

### CASE VIGNETTE 7.1

A 28-year-old active man with type 1 diabetes for 11 years, who attends rarely, wants a medical certificate for driving as he works as a sales rep using a company car all day. He appears fit, weight 71 kg, height 1.73 m, BP 118/74 mmHg and is taking Penmix 30 in a dose of 36 units a.m. and 24 units p.m. He is evasive about his control and own blood tests but the HbA1c is 6.4%; he denies any hypoglycaemia. When you insist, he returns with records that show 15% of readings below 4; he has no clear symptoms with these.

*Comment*

The picture is extremely suggestive of significant hypoglycaemia unawareness, probably due to frequent hypoglycaemia from too tight control. He needs several interventions:[5]

- Education about prevention, recognition and treatment of hypoglycaemia.
- A *significant* reduction in his insulin dose, aimed at avoiding all readings below 4 mmol/l. It is imperative to get rid of *both* 'hypos' *and* readings under 4, even if slight temporary hyperglycaemia results. This is preferable to minor dose reductions with persisting mild hypoglycaemia.
- Over a few months his awareness is likely to improve if he can avoid all hypoglycaemia.
- A review of his insulin regimen, which is not flexible enough and needs to be tailored specifically for him, probably involving multiple injections.
- Education about the rules and precautions for safe driving; he is currently probably unsafe.[12]

These patients are often *very* resistant to advice and require long periods of considerate intervention. Nurse educator and specialist advice is usually needed.

## PERCEPTION, PREVENTION AND TREATMENT OF HYPOGLYCAEMIA

### 7.16  How do patients perceive the risks of hypoglycaemia?

Fear of hypoglycaemia, often unspoken, is a major factor in preventing patients from following advice to aim for tighter control: this relates largely to the embarrassing lack of personal control that hypoglycaemia represents. A single episode that shows the patient as vulnerable and needing help from others can undermine that person's authority or reputation in the eyes of colleagues or friends. Teachers, nurses or those responsible for supervising children or other workers worry greatly about hypoglycaemia and their inability to manage the situation. This leads them 'to run high to be on the safe side'. In type 1 diabetes, this is often their greatest *current* concern and prevents them from following advice on glycaemic control with the *theoretical future risks* of long-term complications.

Patients often feel their physicians are too tolerant of hypoglycaemia.

### 7.17 Are there any other measures to prevent hypoglycaemia?

Much has been covered above but a simple list would be:
- review of the insulin regimen and lifestyle (*see Chapter 6*) and matching insulin to appropriate dietary intake (*see Q. 4.9*)
- checking insulin injection sites, technique and timing
- a larger and more protein-based snack at bedtime on a regular basis
- use of the buttocks as a bedtime injection site to prolong insulin action
- use of an insulin pump in extreme cases, and (very rarely) pancreatic/islet-cell transplantation.

### 7.18 With all the problems of hypoglycaemia, do the benefits of good control outweigh the risks?

Good glycaemic control undoubtedly significantly reduces the long-term risk of microvascular complications. A recent review (*www.clinicalevidence.com*) examined the benefits and risks, concluding that the balance was in favour of good control[13] However, individual patients have a range of views and these need to be explored carefully by the health care professional so that a personal decision is made by each patient.

**PATIENT QUESTION**

### 7.19 How should hypoglycaemia be treated?

With rapidly absorbed glucose, but this is too simple. First hypoglycaemia must be recognised, with confirmation of hypoglycaemia by meter if possible/necessary. Everyone on insulin or sulphonylureas must be taught the risk factors for hypoglycaemia, together with appropriate treatment:

- Immediately eat/drink a *limited* amount of glucose (e.g. two glucose tablets or a small glass of ordinary lemonade).
- Retest blood glucose (if possible/practicable) after 5–10 minutes.
- Eat some longer-acting carbohydrate (e.g. a banana or two biscuits) to maintain blood glucose at safe levels until the next meal.

Afterwards think about why it happened and how similar episodes could be prevented. If it happens frequently or badly, talk to your nurse or doctor.

# Problems with glycaemic control

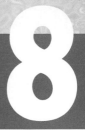

## IDENTIFYING THE PROBLEM

### 8.1 What can be done about people with poorly controlled diabetes?

When faced with a poorly controlled patient, it is vital to identify the reason(s). It is worth explaining that there could be a number of reasons why their control is poor and you need to identify the likely cause(s) so together an attempt can be made to improve matters. A careful history from the patient needs to explore the following main possibilities:
- progressive pancreatic beta-cell failure
- poor compliance with dietary or exercise recommendations
- inadequate doses of prescribed medication
- failure to take prescribed medication regularly
- significant insulin resistance
- emotional stress and psychosocial issues
- other medical illness.

### 8.2 How can I recognise beta-cell failure?

This is probably the commonest cause, though often several factors may be operating. Clues to this include the following:
- The person has had diabetes for some or many years. In general people need insulin after 5–15 years of diagnosed diabetes.
- There has been a progressive requirement for increasing lifestyle intervention and then drug therapy – the UKPDS showed that most patients have a roughly linear rate of deterioration of HbA1c (*see Fig. 2.1*).
- It tends to happen more quickly where patients were more hyperglycaemic at diagnosis (more insulin deficient) than in those with milder hyperglycaemia at presentation.
- Generally insulin is needed earlier in younger patients of normal weight.
 Insulin should be presented positively as the treatment of choice (*see Q. 6.9*), not as the only option left. The eventual need is best discussed years before it is needed (*see Q. 6.7*).

### 8.3 How do you find out if dietary indiscretion is responsible?

This can be difficult. Asking a partner to join in the discussion is often helpful. One useful approach is to say: 'No one with diabetes is perfect on the diet. What are your weaknesses?', then gently explore how often/how much they eat those foods while commending areas of success.

■ A general discussion of food intake will help you estimate if this is a significant cause of the problem.

■ Quantity is often the issue. They may only eat 'healthy recommended foods' but portion sizes may be massive. A clue to this is when weight continues to increase despite poor glycaemic control.

■ Alcohol intake (and associated 'mixers') may be a major factor. Low sugar soft drinks are often not available in many bars and pubs.

Dietary referral is often helpful but it is critical to involve the patient and not just 'pass the buck' to the dietitian! Self-motivation is essential.

### 8.4 The reason for poor glycaemic control is failure to stick to the diet. Should I increase the medication?

There is no straightforward answer here. In the real world few, if any, people with diabetes can realistically eat healthily all the time. Nor does 100% compliance with diet guarantee good control – the natural history of pancreatic failure will eventually win!

Leaving patients poorly controlled is no longer acceptable when safe therapy, especially metformin, carries no significant adverse risk. A pragmatic approach is firstly to try to help the patient understand the problem and then to use medication carefully.

In overweight/obese patients metformin should be used to maximum doses if tolerated and not contraindicated. It does not lead to weight gain, is helpful in insulin resistance and may improve glycaemic control, possibly due to the side effects of slight anorexia and consequent reduced food intake! (*See also Case vignettes 5.4 and 5.5.*)

All other treatments for diabetes tend to increase weight. Insulin therapy and insulin secretagogues also carry the risk of hypoglycaemia. It is easy to start a vicious circle of increasing medication, appetite, weight gain and worsening poor control. In the insulin-treated patient with type 2 diabetes, continually increasing insulin doses (especially above 1 unit/kg) is often unproductive. Specialist advice is often needed with these difficult cases to ensure that everything possible is being tried.

### 8.5 What clues are there to suggest that insufficient therapy is the cause of poor glycaemic control?

The best clue is to review the control over the past few visits.

■ In the first year after diagnosis, if good control has never been achieved and dietary/exercise compliance has been reasonable, then probably insufficient OHAs have been prescribed.

■ Some people make a rapid transition through maximal medication to need insulin. This is commoner if HbA1c is very high at diagnosis and/or complications are already present, suggesting a long period of undiagnosed hyperglycaemia.

■ When there is steady deterioration of HbA1c with stable weight, then deteriorating beta-cell function is likely and OHA treatment should be increased. In general, starting metformin or a sulphonylurea leads to a reduction in HbA1c of 1–2% but, with increasing dose, the response is less, due to flattening of the dose–response curve and a failing pancreas.

Now that glycaemic control targets have been tightened, you may find patients where control has never been good and treatment was not optimised. Patients find this hard to understand and it is important to explain why you are now advocating more intensive treatment. (*See also Case vignettes 5.4 and 5.5.*)

## 8.6 How about adherence?

Poor compliance with or adherence to prescribed oral and insulin medication is very common (*see Case vignettes 5.4, 5.5 and 8.1*). The DART study in Scotland monitored prescription encashment at the pharmacy and found that most people with diabetes do not obtain as much medication as is prescribed, suggesting doses are frequently missed. The more treatments prescribed and more frequent dosing positively correlated with worsening compliance.[1]

In primary care it should be possible to review the frequency of repeat prescription requests to gain some idea of compliance. Trying to simplify the medication schedule can be helpful:

■ Using once-daily long-acting preparations where possible, avoiding a lunchtime dose when possible.
■ Using combined tablets where available.
■ Sticking to twice-daily rather than three-times daily dosing is often helpful (e.g. metformin 850 mg + 1700 mg rather than 850 mg t.d.s.).
■ Make quite clear to the patient what each medication is for.

## 8.7 Is the dose of insulin adequate? Or is the cause insulin resistance?

*Adequate insulin*

For insulin-treated patients, it is worth calculating the dose in units/kg body weight. Those of normal weight will generally be well controlled when insulin doses are ≤ 1.0 unit/kg, except in puberty when changing hormones lead to increasing insulin requirement up to 1.5 units/kg.

If the dosage is much higher and the HbA1c is >11% in a patient with a BMI below 25, then missed insulin doses are likely. This is commonly seen in teenagers and young adults, but also occurs in others (e.g. the elderly when memory is poor). It is not worth increasing the insulin dose, as they still won't take it regularly (or become hypoglycaemic when they do!), but simplification of the regimen may help. Teenagers rarely admit their insulin omission at the time, but often do so years later! (*See also Case vignette 8.4.*)

Injection technique or faulty pen devices can sometimes be behind poor control. Frequent injection into areas of lipohypertrophy can lead to erratic absorption. Checking injection sites is important and often neglected; a review by a diabetes nurse specialist is often valuable in uncovering problems.

### Insulin resistance

Patients with insulin resistance[2] are usually obese and have features of the metabolic syndrome such as hypertension, hyperlipidaemia and a high waist circumference (*see Box 1.3*). They frequently undertake little exercise and fail to lose weight despite encouragement. Metformin and/or glitazones (TZDs) are preferable in this group. When these fail to adequately control glucose levels, sulphonylurea treatment can be tried but such patients often end up on insulin in surprisingly large doses: 1–1.5 units/kg. With larger doses of insulin (above a single dose of 50–60 units), splitting the injection into two smaller doses may help to improve absorption. However, if progressively increasing doses fail to improve control, then consider asking for specialist advice. This is a difficult group of patients as there can develop a vicious circle of increasing weight and insulin doses – the 'insulin sink' syndrome (*see also Q. 6.16*).

---

### 8.8 Can stress really cause poor glycaemic control?

Yes. This can be easily recognised in some patients where control has been satisfactory for some time, but when a significant life event occurs control rapidly worsens. If the event is short lived, stable good control may return but sometimes, despite resolution of the problem, control remains poor and treatment needs to be increased. One can speculate that the period of hyperglycaemia leads to more rapid beta-cell deterioration. The problem can be caused by an acute physical illness (e.g. influenza) as well as mental stress (*see Case vignette 8.4*).[3]

It is more difficult to detect this soon after diagnosis unless the patient is well known to you. For some the diagnosis of diabetes is itself the stressor and, as the patient struggles to cope emotionally with the problem, glucose levels remain high or swing rapidly. This situation is seen in a few people with type 1 diabetes and their anxiety and desperate desire to control their blood glucose (BG) levels lead to persistently high BG levels or wildly fluctuating control. It is only when they relax their efforts or begin to put diabetes management into perspective that control seems to improve. Psychological help may be valuable for these individuals.[4]

Occasionally, but not often, occult physical illness is the underlying cause of deterioration of glycaemic control. If there seems to be no obvious reason why glycaemic control has worsened, a full history, examination and simple investigations may be worthwhile.

## BEHAVIOURAL ISSUES

### 8.9 How do I persuade and motivate patients to achieve better control of their diabetes?

Improved control of diabetes usually only occurs when it nears the top of the patient's agenda. A recent study (DAWN – diabetes, attitudes, wishes and needs) has shed some light on the importance of social support and emotional well-being in achieving effective self-management (*www.dawnstudy.com*).

These are issues which apply to many illnesses, and diabetes only differs in its permanent nature and the enormous extent of personal involvement required every day. They include the patient's relationships, outlook on life and daily stresses.[5] Particular problems are anger and resentment about diabetes, denial and lack of understanding (*see Case vignette 7.1*). Fear of complications rarely produces a positive response.

### 8.10 The results of the patient's home monitoring don't seem to agree with the laboratory HbA1c. What should I do?

This is common and the possible causes should be explored. Often the simple discrepancy should just be pointed out to the patient, and possible causes enumerated:

- The equipment used for BG self-monitoring may be old, not working properly or not being used correctly.
- If home urine testing is being undertaken, the patient may have a high renal threshold for glucose – compare the laboratory glucose with a simultaneous urine test.
- Sometimes only fasting or pre-prandial BGs are done, with large post-prandial rises being the issue.

Usually, however, technical issues are not the real problem. Patients generally want to please and show their diabetes is well controlled. Some find it difficult to monitor their diabetes at the frequency suggested and 'invent' some or all of their results – beware the tidy book with neat figures and no blood or coffee stains! Alternatively, they may only record 'good' tests. These situations need to be approached with sensitivity. Most modern meters have a memory recording results, time and date, sometimes also calculating an average. Checking this can give an idea of these results and how they tally with the diary.

Some patients will only record results for the 2 weeks before a visit. When HbA1c and BGs don't agree, one suspects this may be the only time when diabetes care is taken seriously! Many patients and professionals fail to recognise that home monitoring is *for the patient's use, not just the doctor's*. Patients should be encouraged to bring home monitoring results to consultations; carers should examine them carefully, discuss their significance and help people to adjust their treatment and/or to be confident that their control is satisfactory.

## ACHIEVING TARGETS FOR GLYCAEMIC CONTROL

### 8.11 I can't seem to get my newly diagnosed patient adequately controlled by lifestyle measures. How long should I persist before introducing oral agents?

This has been largely dealt with in *Questions 3.18 and 5.1*, and illustrative examples are given in *Case vignettes 5.1–5.3*.

### 8.12 When should a patient on maximum OHAs be changed to insulin treatment?

This has been considered in *Question 6.7*, and illustrative examples are given in *Case vignettes 5.4, 5.5 and 8.1–8.3*.

### 8.13 Not many of my patients seem to reach desirable glycaemic targets. What can I do to improve this situation?

Do your patients know or understand the targets you are both working towards? Surprisingly many patients are ignorant of these. Two randomised studies in type 2 diabetes showed that education about glycaemic targets led to significantly improved control over 4 years. One study in Italy achieved this through group education sessions and the other in Israel through a single 90-minute individual education session.[6,7]

Helping people to understand can be a crucial factor: the patient-held record book is a useful tool where targets are written and results are entered at each visit. Copying the laboratory results for the patients can also help understanding and self-involvement.

## 8.14 Are there any new guidelines for type 1 diabetes?

In 2004, NICE published guidelines for management of type 1 diabetes covering a wide range of topics and based on the most up to date evidence available. As well as a summary reference guide for professionals, a special version is available for people with type 1 diabetes. Advice about glycaemic control includes a general recommendation to aim for HbA1c <7.5% to minimise the risk of long-term complications. Home blood glucose monitoring targets are 4–7 mmol/l before meals and <9 mmol/l after meals for adults, with a more flexible range for children of 4–8 mmol/l before meals and <10 mmol/l after meals.

## CASE VIGNETTES IN POOR GLYCAEMIC CONTROL

### CASE VIGNETTE 8.1

A 62-year-old woman has had type 2 diabetes for 7 years and hypertension for 3 years; BMI is 34 kg/m$^2$. Despite metformin 850 mg t.d.s. and gliclazide modified release 120 mg daily, fasting glucose is 9.5 mmol/l, HbA1c 8.7% and creatinine 78 µmol/l.

*Comment*

The glycaemic control is suboptimal but she is already on maximal combination treatment. Diet and exercise have presumably already been exhausted as possible options, as she is significantly overweight. The next step in intervention includes insulin or a thiazolidinedione: a night-time dose of long-acting insulin with continuation of metformin may improve glycaemic control but may produce significant weight gain; the alternative is to use a thiazolidinedione though this will also cause weight gain.

In the UK, the prescribing licence for TZDs is in combination with either metformin or a sulphonylurea, *not* as triple combination therapy. In an overweight patient, you might consider a switch from gliclazide to rosiglitazone or pioglitazone. However, this may lead to a rapid deterioration in control within a few days before the TZD becomes effective over several months. In addition, the HbA1c response to TZDs will probably only be similar to that seen with the gliclazide. Increasingly, specialists are prescribing triple therapy in this situation after informing the patient that this is outside the current prescribing licence and that hard evidence is still awaited. In the USA, triple therapy is licensed. It does appear, however, that – both clinically and economically – this is not often superior to insulin and it would be worth consulting with a specialist before taking this step. (Note: gliclazide MR 120 mg daily is equivalent to gliclazide 160 mg b.d.)

### CASE VIGNETTE 8.2

After a hospital admission for angina, a 69-year-old woman with type 2 diabetes, hypertension and mild dyslipidaemia for 10 years remains overweight. Treatment is metformin 850 mg b.d. and gliclazide modified release 120 mg daily. Fasting glucose is 10.1 mmol/l, HbA1c 8.7% and creatinine 86 µmol/l.

*Comment*

Again, glycaemic control is not ideal. Considering the discussion in Case 8.1, the addition of a TZD or nocturnal insulin might be considered as the next step. However, caution is required when used with insulin – in one study 2.5% of patients on insulin and TZDs developed heart failure. This may relate to the common side effect of fluid retention but, in a patient with a history of angina, caution is recommended.

The DIGAMI trial[8] – where intensive insulin therapy was used immediately after an acute myocardial infarction in patients with diabetes and continued for at least 3 months – showed a substantial and significant reduction in mortality. Though there is no acute myocardial infarction, she clearly has coronary artery disease: earlier use of insulin should be considered more often in these patients.

Addition of nocturnal basal insulin to improve fasting PG levels might be particularly helpful as these levels are significantly raised. But insulin may also result in 2–3 kg weight gain, possibly aggravating angina symptoms and worsening hypertension control. This is a difficult decision and can only be resolved by considering all the medical and lifestyle issues together with patient preference and probably a specialist opinion.

## CASE VIGNETTE 8.3

A 73-year-old overweight man with 11 years of diabetes on maximal oral agents is becoming progressively poorly controlled on maximal glipizide and metformin with fasting glucose 11.4 mmol/l, HbA1c 10.3%. Renal function is normal.

*Comment*

Glycaemic control is unacceptable. Addition of a TZD as triple therapy is most unlikely to achieve the desired 2–3% reduction in HbA1c, and he needs insulin treatment. Whilst once daily or nocturnal long-acting insulin combined with his OHAs is tempting, he probably has too little residual beta-cell function for this to work. Assuming there are no major dietary or exercise issues (unlikely), he needs full insulinisation with continuation of the metformin to reduce insulin dose and control his weight. Possible options are:

- ■ Twice-daily isophane, with a later change to a pre-mixed insulin or complex regimen if post prandial BGs remain high.
- ■ A standard twice-daily pre-mixed insulin (e.g. Novomix 30) is likely to be effective.

The metformin in this situation may minimise the weight gain with insulin, and allow 15–20% smaller doses of insulin to be effective.

## CASE VIGNETTE 8.4

An apparently fit young woman of 22 has had type 1 diabetes for 2 years. She weighs 52 kg with a BMI of 21.3 kg/m². Her current treatment is Mixtard 30 insulin 42 units twice daily but doses have gradually increased over the last year and HbA1c remains extremely high at 12.4%. What is the best way to improve control?

*Comment*

She is on a large dose of insulin for her size, 1.6 units/kg, even for post-adolescence, so simply increasing the insulin dose is unlikely to improve her control. The HbA1c suggests her PG levels are mostly around 15 mmol/l. The likeliest causes, of which more than one may be relevant, are:

- ■ stress and emotion
- ■ insulin omission
- ■ poor diet
- ■ physical illness.

Emotional issues, stress and adjustment to the diagnosis of diabetes are common. People going through difficult personal circumstances can show tremendous swings in BG levels (*see Q. 8.8*). She may not have come to terms with her diabetes, even though this was 2 years ago.

Insulin omission and a poor diet are common in this young adult group. Tackling these issues can be difficult. It is generally pointless to ask directly about omission as the patient is forced into a corner with denial. Exploring whether the insulin regimen suits them, or whether they have a needle phobia and using a device to help to inject might be an option. A potential problem here is that the insulin dose is really too high. So, if and when she *does* comply with correct diet and frequency of injections, hypoglycaemia may occur – thus reinforcing her anxieties. Discussing a more realistic insulin dose can be valuable. The final problem to recognise is that many young women use poor control of their diabetes to control their weight – eating disorders including bulimia are commoner in this group.[9]

Physical illness can occasionally lead to insulin resistance. History and examination can exclude more obvious causes but, rarely, occult disease can be more difficult to identify. Assessment by a diabetes nurse specialist and possibly a psychologist might be very helpful, before a physician review.

# Decompensated diabetes

# 9

## ACUTE ILLNESS IN PEOPLE WITH DIABETES

### 9.1 What advice should be given to people with diabetes when they are ill?

Surprisingly, many people with diabetes are unaware that physical or mental illness can lead to raised or variable blood glucose (BG) levels, partly due to increased stress hormones such as cortisol and adrenaline which impair the glucose response to insulin. Even a trivial upper respiratory tract infection can cause this.

Patients should monitor their diabetes more closely during illness. Those used to adjusting treatment should be encouraged to do so if BG levels rise. Telephone advice needs to be readily available so that individualised recommendations can be made – most diabetes services will provide this, at least during the working week.

Good educational materials ('Sick day rules') can be found on many patient-orientated websites, including material that can be printed out (*www.diabetes.org.uk*). A summary is shown in *Box 9.1*.

---

**BOX 9.1  Sick day rules**

During illness or infection your blood glucose can often rise even though you are not eating as much as normal:

- *Test your blood glucose more often than normal*: about four times a day is sensible; if levels are continuing to rise despite the advice below, contact your GP or diabetes team.

- *Never stop or reduce taking your insulin or tablets without medical advice*: this is the commonest mistake made. In this situation the body often needs more insulin, not less.

- *If you cannot eat normally, substitute meals with simple foods*, such as:
  — soups and bread
  — milk pudding, custard or yoghurt
  — breakfast cereals and milk.

- *If you can only manage fluids, sip one of the following every 2 hours or so*:
  — a glass of ordinary lemonade (not 'diet')
  — a glass of fruit juice (e.g. orange or apple).

- *An adequate fluid intake is vital*: you need at least 3 litres of fluids daily – water is the best additional one. If you cannot maintain this, or are vomiting or have severe diarrhoea, then get medical help quickly.

- *If things aren't getting better quickly, call for help*: your GP is there to help, and many diabetes centres run telephone helplines.

BOX 9.1 (*Cont'd*) Sick day rules

For patients with type 1 diabetes:

- You may also need to test your urine for ketones if you know how.
- You may need additional doses of short-acting insulin if glucoses are over 10–15 mmol/l.
- If you have more than two readings over 20 mmol/l then get help.

## 9.2    When do people with diabetes need hospital admission?

Decompensated diabetes can lead to serious consequences such as diabetic ketoacidosis (DKA) and hyperosmolar non-ketotic coma (HONK). Recognising the onset of these conditions is not always easy and knowing the patient's previous medical history, particularly the prior level of glycaemic control, is helpful. Children with type 1 diabetes or older patients who have been poorly controlled can deteriorate within a few hours.

Dehydration or persistent vomiting always necessitates hospital admission, and high BG levels (i.e. > 30 mmol/l) are always of concern. It may be possible to manage the latter without admission by giving a dose of quick-acting insulin if the patient is well hydrated, not vomiting and with good social support, but a follow-up call to ensure recovery is critical. Lower BG levels can occasionally be deceptive if the patient has continued with insulin or even increased doses, as ketoacidosis can still develop. Look for signs of acidosis such as tachypnoea: if in doubt emergency department assessment is wise (*see Case vignette 9.1*).

Patients treated with an insulin pump can deteriorate very rapidly and dangerous hyperkalaemia can develop within a few hours. Such patients do not have a subcutaneous reservoir of insulin in their body as do those using conventional injections, and so hyperglycaemia with metabolic decompensation occurs rapidly. Blocked cannulae or infection at the subcutaneous infusion site can be causes and need to be treated seriously.

In type 2 diabetes, HONK usually develops over a period of days. The gradual deterioration and lack of vomiting often leads to a delay in the diagnosis. It can occur in patients previously undiagnosed or treated with diet alone or relatively low doses of oral hypoglycaemic agents (OHAs). Confusion is common and an infection is the usual triggering event. BG levels are commonly >50 mmol/l but ketoacidosis does not occur because the patient continues to secrete low levels of insulin, sufficient to prevent fat breakdown but inadequate to control hyperglycaemia.

**CASE VIGNETTE 9.1**

A 28-year-old man with type 1 diabetes for 6 years phones for advice. He has been vomiting for 4 hours since breakfast. He is on short-acting insulin before each meal and long-acting insulin at night. His BG has risen from 9 to 16 mmol/l. What should be done about his diabetes management?

*Comment*

Obviously, you need to be clear about how unwell he is, what other symptoms are present and whether there is a clear underlying diagnosis. A home/surgery assessment is necessary if there are worrying features such as fever and rigors, or if there is little social support. It is critical that he continues to administer his insulin even though he is unable to eat any food. As his BG is rising, you might advise an extra 2–6 units with his lunchtime dose and to take frequent sips of a sugary drink if unable to eat.

If vomiting is due to a minor episode of gastroenteritis, the patient may remain at home taking fluids, extra insulin and possibly an anti-emetic injection. However, he will need to know when to call for further help – certainly persistent vomiting for 6–8 hours is likely to lead to dehydration and ketoacidosis. Follow-up phone calls to check progress in a few hours and before bedtime are essential.

If his glycaemic control is generally poor or his ability to cope is in doubt (e.g. if he lives alone), early hospital admission is preferable.

### 9.3 When called to see an unconscious diabetic patient, how can you differentiate between hyper- and hypoglycaemia?

This is usually obvious from the history and circumstances, if necessary gleaned from witnesses. Rapid onset within minutes always suggests hypoglycaemia. If the patient has been found in bed comatose, hypoglycaemia is likely if the patient was well the night before (*see Case vignette 9.2*).

When no history is available, measuring a fingerprick BG should differentiate between the two conditions but, if this is unavailable, then other symptoms and signs are helpful (*Table 9.1*). If hypoglycaemia is suspected, a sample for later laboratory plasma glucose (PG) estimation is valuable. If there remains doubt it is worth treating for hypoglycaemia (*see Q. 9.4*) as little harm can be done.

Finally, always bear in mind that other causes of coma are always possible in someone with diabetes (e.g. overdose, stroke) (*see Case vignette 9.3*).

**TABLE 9.1 The common differentiating features between hypoglycaemia and hyperglycaemia**

|  | Hypoglycaemia | Hyperglycaemia |
|---|---|---|
| Onset | Rapid (within minutes) | Gradual (over many hours) |
| Hydration | Normal | Dehydrated |
| Breathing | Normal | Rapid |
| Seizures | Common | Uncommon |
| Perspiration | Heavy sweating | None unless feverish due to infection |

## CASE VIGNETTE 9.2

A 20-year-old man with type 1 diabetes has been found unconscious in bed in the students' residence at 10 a.m. He is unrousable but his BG is normal at 7.4 mmol/l.

*Comment*

Assuming there is no other pathology such as dehydration and vomiting, head injury or drug/alcohol overdose, he has probably suffered an episode of severe nocturnal hypoglycaemia. The stress response to prolonged neuroglycopenia eventually leads to cortisol and adrenaline secretion which in turn increase PG levels.

He needs urgent transfer to hospital for full assessment. In most cases, the brain injury is transient and recovery occurs over hours or days during which he may be confused. However, a few cases develop permanent brain damage and never make a full recovery. Very rarely patients are actually found 'dead in bed' – presumed but not proven to have suffered a severe hypoglycaemic attack and possibly a cardiac dysrhythmia.

Alcohol and possibly drugs may be risk factors for nocturnal hypoglycaemia. Alcohol tends to increase the risk of hypoglycaemia by impairing hepatic glucose release from the liver as well as masking early symptoms.

## CASE VIGNETTE 9.3

A 76-year-old man with type 2 diabetes usually has excellent glycaemic control, HbA1c 6.6%, on glibenclamide 10 mg daily. His daughter found him on the floor with right-sided weakness and unable to talk. She reports that he had not felt well the day before with fever, nausea and abdominal discomfort.

*Comment*

At first sight, you may suspect a stroke producing a right-sided hemiplegia with aphasia, but he may be suffering from hypoglycaemia causing the neurological deficit. He needs a fingerprick BG sample checked and if this is <4 mmol/l, a sugary drink (if the swallowing reflex is intact) or intravenous glucose should be administered (*see Q. 9.4*). He is usually well controlled and if he has taken insufficient food, hypoglycaemia can occur.

Glucose meters are useful here but not infallible – a common error is for sugary food to have contaminated the fingers and so overestimate BG.

The nausea and abdominal discomfort might be caused by a urinary tract infection, with deterioration in renal function leading to accumulation of glibenclamide and a substantial risk of hypoglycaemia. He needs hospital admission – as do all patients suffering significant hypoglycaemia from sulphonylurea as the hypoglycaemia can be very prolonged and severe during the subsequent 24–36 hours and carries a significant risk of morbidity and mortality.

---

### 9.4 What is the best treatment for hypoglycaemia when the patient is comatose?

- ■ Intravenous dextrose 50% 20–50 ml, or 50–100 ml of 10–20% dextrose (the 50% formulation is very corrosive to veins and tissues).
- ■ Intramuscular glucagon 1 mg is an alternative if intravenous access is difficult, but takes 10–15 minutes to work and often causes vomiting.
- ■ Buccal dextrose gel (e.g. Hypostop), provided swallowing reflex and airway protection are intact.

> Once patients have recovered, they must always be encouraged to eat a carbohydrate snack to prevent recurrence of the hypoglycaemia – the half-life of intravenous or buccal glucose is only a few minutes.
>
> If the episode has been induced by sulphonylurea treatment, hospital assessment is needed as recurrent severe hypoglycaemia is common, especially with glibenclamide.
>
> After a severe 'hypo' it is important to establish the precipitating factor(s) so they can be avoided in future (*see Ch. 7*).

## STEROIDS AND DIABETES

### 9.5 How do steroids affect glycaemic control in diabetes?

 Steroids impair the glucose response to insulin leading to an increase in insulin resistance and consequently increase PG levels. A short course of steroid (or steroid injection for musculoskeletal problems) will lead to derangement of BGs for a few days only. The response will depend on previous glycaemic control and the dose of steroid used. People need to understand the likely deterioration in control and be advised to monitor more closely for a few days.

Patients often report that steroids were not prescribed because of their diabetes. The indication for steroid treatment needs to be carefully considered, but if the condition warrants such treatment then the steroid should be prescribed and not withheld – diabetes treatment can be adjusted to cope with steroid treatment.

### 9.6 How should diabetes be managed when a patient needs a short course of steroids (e.g. for worsening asthma)?

In these situations steroids are usually given at high dose (e.g. prednisolone 30 mg daily, for 7–10 days). More frequent monitoring should be recommended and patients warned about the probable effect on BG. If on diet alone, no action may be needed if preceding control has been reasonably good. For those on OHAs or insulin, it is common to need a temporary increase in dose. The advice should be individualised according to pre-existing treatment and control.

With a single morning dose of steroid, BG levels usually rise predominantly during the afternoon until bedtime. By next morning, they have often returned to reasonable levels. For patients on twice-daily insulins, increased morning doses are usually needed, often substantially more (*see Case vignette 9.4*).

**CASE VIGNETTE 9.4**

A 72-year-old lady with type 2 diabetes also now has temporal arteritis and has started prednisolone 30 mg daily; the headaches disappeared completely within a few days. However, she is now feeling thirsty with nocturia three times per night. She was previously well controlled with gliclazide 160 mg twice daily and metformin 500 mg twice daily. A random BG is 23 mmol/l.

*Comment*

Patients treated with steroids for conditions such as temporal arteritis, polymyalgia rheumatica or vasculitis are usually on reducing doses of steroids for many months and, possibly, years. Prednisolone in a dose above 5 mg daily is likely to affect glycaemic control: the higher the dose the greater the effect. She now has marked symptoms of hyperglycaemia and increasing the dose of metformin is unlikely to control this; she will need insulin.

Highest BG levels are usually seen in the late afternoon and evening. To achieve optimal control, a multiple insulin injection therapy would probably be required. However, given her age, her other medical problems and the variable steroid dose, such intensive treatment may not be appropriate. A reasonable compromise would be twice-daily pre-mixed insulin such as Mixtard 30 – the greater dose will be needed in the morning. This should lead to adequate control and improve the symptoms relating to hyperglycaemia; if this fails a more intensive regimen might be used.

The insulin dose will need reducing as the steroid dose comes down, and a careful watch for overnight hypoglycaemia will be necessary – often only once-daily morning insulin is needed at lower doses of prednisolone.

---

**9.7   How is diabetes managed when a patient is being starved for an investigation or procedure such as a gastroscopy?**

Most endoscopy and day surgical units have guidelines to advise patients and clinicians on how to manage diabetes. It is important that any referral includes information relating to diabetes and its treatment.

■ For patients on diet alone or on metformin, fasting will not lead to hypoglycaemia.

■ Patients treated with insulin or sulphonylureas may experience hypoglycaemia if fasting is prolonged.

■ Usually, people with diabetes have their procedure at the beginning of the morning or afternoon so fasting is minimised.

■ If undertaken in the morning, insulin or OHAs can be delayed until after the procedure. The dose of insulin may need to be reduced for those on the afternoon list.

■ For people on twice-daily insulin, we advise giving half their usual morning dose before breakfast and fasting from mid-morning. If treated with short-acting insulin before meals and long-acting insulin at bedtime, the lunchtime dose can be delayed until after the procedure.

The endoscopy/anaesthetic nurse should check the BG before and after the procedure to make sure there is no hypoglycaemia.

Patients undergoing a colonoscopy will be prepared for the procedure by changing their diet and having extensive laxatives. During this time, the patient treated with insulin or OHAs may experience hypoglycaemia if insufficient food is taken. Supplements of sugary drinks and dose reductions may be required.

Patients should be warned that that the stress of such procedures may upset BG levels for a while.

## INPATIENT MANAGEMENT OF DIABETES

### 9.8 Why is diabetic control upset when a patient is admitted to hospital?

Most people with diabetes notice deterioration in glycaemic control when admitted to hospital. This is easily understood when one considers the changes that occur at this time. The patient's routine is disturbed and normal activity is probably markedly curtailed, food provided in hospital is often different in quantity, quality and timing and the physical and emotional stress of being admitted to hospital will itself lead to increased BG concentrations (*see Q. 8.8*). The only factor likely to reduce BG levels is poor appetite and food intake!

### 9.9 Does good glycaemic control matter when having surgery?

Yes. There is evidence from many different branches of surgery that poor glycaemic control in people with diabetes is associated with poorer outcomes, higher infection and complication rates and longer hospital stays.[1]

With ever-decreasing times between admission and surgery, especially day cases, poor glycaemic control is a major cause of delayed or cancelled surgery. Patients on waiting lists should have their control improved urgently or, if indications for surgery are urgent, an insulin infusion should be used to cover the period of surgery. Good liaison and communication between primary and secondary care is vital here.

Most hospitals have defined local protocols for management of diabetes during surgery.

### 9.10 What can be done to improve diabetes control in hospital?

Monitoring BG levels regularly when in hospital is crucial. This needs to be combined with appropriate adjustment of diabetes treatment. A well-educated patient with diabetes can and should continue their own self-management in hospital, provided staff discuss the planned investigations and treatment. Diabetologists often give patients a letter to recommend continuing self-management, which is usually copied to the consultant/unit responsible for the admission.

When patients need modification of their treatment during admissions, specialist diabetes teams are usually available to advise. One common error from non-specialist teams is the use of subcutaneous insulin 'sliding scales' which have no scientific backing.

Following discharge and return to normal activities, careful monitoring and treatment adjustment are often needed.

### 9.11 Is there a problem with the use of metformin and X-ray investigations?

Radiological contrast material can cause serious deterioration in renal function in people with diabetes, this then being a contraindication to metformin and a risk factor for lactic acidosis (*see Q. 5.7*).[2] This has resulted in strict guidelines – contrast will normally only be administered if metformin has been withdrawn 24 hours before any such procedure, and withheld for 48 hours afterwards. Contrast material is also frequently given for CT or MRI scanning and obviously in all forms of angiography. X-ray request forms should *always* include the diagnosis of diabetes (and its treatment) to avoid potential problems or late cancellations. A recent report suggests that new iso-osmolar contrast agents may prevent this problem, but they are not yet in widespread use.

**PATIENT QUESTION**

**9.12 What should I do if I'm unwell?**

This is important and is summarised in *Box 9.1*. Further details are available in patient leaflets and from websites, such as *www.diabetes.org.uk.*

# Organisation and delivery of diabetes care

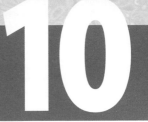

## NATIONAL STANDARDS FOR DIABETES AND THE CARE TEAM

### 10.1 What is the National Service Framework for Diabetes?

The NHS has developed national service frameworks (NSFs) for several diseases such as cancer, and for patient groups such as the elderly. They have used external reference groups that include experts in the field, representatives of all groups of health professionals, patients and health service managers. The first document for diabetes in 2001 set a framework for care by including standards, rationales, key interventions and an analysis of the implications for planning services.[1] It was followed in 2002 by 'The Delivery Strategy', which sets out how it should be implemented over a 10-year period.[2]

Many countries have undertaken similar exercises, which help to set standards of care for people with diabetes. It is well recognised that everyone should receive regular and systematic care, irrespective of where they live or who provides it.

*Table 10.1* gives a concise summary of the National Service Framework for Diabetes (*www.doh.gov.uk/nsf/diabetes*).

| TABLE 10.1  National Service Framework for Diabetes: standards[1] | |
| --- | --- |
| **Framework** | **Standard summary** |
| Prevention of type 2 diabetes | *Standard 1*: The NHS will develop, implement and monitor strategies to reduce the risk of developing type 2 diabetes in the population as a whole and to reduce the inequalities in the risk of developing type 2 diabetes. |
| Identification of people with diabetes | *Standard 2*: The NHS will develop, implement and monitor strategies to identify people who do not know they have diabetes. |
| Empowering people with diabetes | *Standard 3*: All children, young people and adults with diabetes will receive a service which encourages partnership in decision making, supports them in managing their diabetes and helps them to adopt and maintain a healthy lifestyle. This will be reflected in an agreed and shared care plan in an appropriate format and language. Where appropriate, parents and carers should be fully engaged in this process. |
| Clinical care of adults with diabetes | *Standard 4*: All adults with diabetes will receive high-quality care throughout their lifetime, including support to optimise the control of their blood glucose, blood pressure and other risk factors for developing the complications of diabetes. |

**TABLE 10.1 (Cont'd) National Service Framework for Diabetes: standards[1]**

| Framework | Standard summary |
| --- | --- |
| Clinical care of children and young people with diabetes | *Standard 5*: All children and young people with diabetes will receive consistently high-quality care and they, with their families and others involved in their day-to-day care, will be supported to optimise the control of their blood glucose and their physical, psychological, intellectual, educational and social development. *Standard 6*: All young people with diabetes will experience a smooth transition of care from paediatric diabetes services to adult diabetes services, whether hospital- or community-based, either directly or via a young people's clinic. The transition will be organised in partnership with each individual and at an age appropriate to and agreed with them. |
| Management of diabetic emergencies | *Standard 7*: The NHS will develop, implement and monitor agreed protocols for rapid and effective treatment of diabetic emergencies by appropriately trained health care professionals. Protocols will include the management of acute complications and procedures to minimise the risk of recurrence. |
| Care of people with diabetes during admission to hospital | *Standard 8*: All children, young people and adults with diabetes admitted to hospital, for whatever reason, will receive effective care of their diabetes. Wherever possible, they will continue to be involved in decisions concerning the management of their diabetes. |
| Diabetes and pregnancy | *Standard 9*: The NHS will develop, implement and monitor policies that seek to empower and support women with pre-existing diabetes and those who develop diabetes during pregnancy to optimise the outcomes of their pregnancy. |
| Detection and management of long-term complications (Standards 10–12) | *Standard 10*: All young people and adults with diabetes will receive regular surveillance for the long-term complications of diabetes. *Standard 11*: The NHS will develop, implement and monitor agreed protocols and systems of care to ensure that all people who develop long-term complications of diabetes receive timely, appropriate and effective investigation and treatment to reduce their risk of disability and premature death. *Standard 12*: All people with diabetes requiring multi-agency support will receive integrated health and social care. |

## 10.2 Who should be involved in the diabetes care team?

Optimal diabetes care is a team effort, perhaps more so than any other area of medicine. It requires skills from a wide range of individuals and departments, and should centre around the person with diabetes.[3,4]

Special mention should be made of diabetes nurse specialists/nurse educators. These roles were developed over 20 years ago (often cited as the first example of a specialist nursing role) and they form the backbone of many services. Apart from a high-quality specialist education in clinical diabetes, they are also trained and skilled in educational methods.

It is always worth remembering that many patients with diabetes have more relevant knowledge than junior or younger members of the team and, sometimes, than their seniors! They do not take kindly to uninformed advice!

## 10.3 How can I be sure that I provide a good standard of diabetes care in my practice?

It is easy to make presumptions about diabetes care but the only real test is to systematically measure some main aspects:
- Appropriate screening for and detection of diabetes
- The processes of care
- The outcomes of care
- Patient satisfaction with care.

The first level of audit is to ensure that the actual processes of care are being undertaken (*Table 10.2*). Ideally 100% of patients should have each procedure undertaken but it is extremely difficult to fulfil this standard. It can be demoralising to set a target too high and constantly fail. A good practice should be able to achieve most standards in 85–90% of patients. If starting from a low baseline, try setting the standard at 50% the first year, 65% in the second and 80% in the third to make an achievable goal.

Once you have set your own practice standards, undertake the audit on either all the records of people with diabetes or a random sample if the practice is large. Review the results and investigate why the standard is not being reached.

In the UK, the new General Medical Services (GMS) GP contract has set quality indicators for diabetes care which are now the important audit standards.

**TABLE 10.2  An abbreviated summary of GMS contract indicators (and useful audit measures) for diabetes***

| Indicator | Measure (abbreviated) | Points | Target |
|---|---|---|---|
| 1 | Practice can produce a register of all patients with diabetes[†] | 6 | Yes! |
| 2 | Percentage of patients with diabetes mellitus with BMI in notes in last 12 months | 3 | 90% |
| 3 | Percentage of patients with smoking status recorded (or those recorded as 'never' smokers) | 3 | 90% |
| 4 | Percentage of smoking patients offered cessation advice in that time | 5 | 90% |
| 5 | Percentage of patients with record of HbA1c | 3 | 90% |
| 6 | Percentage of these patients with HbA1c ≤7.4% | 16 | 50% |
| 7 | Percentage of these patients with HbA1c ≤10% | 11 | 85% |
| 8 | Percentage of patients with a record of retinal screening | 5 | 90% |
| 9 | Percentage of patients with a record of peripheral pulses | 3 | 90% |
| 10 | Percentage of patients with a record of neuropathy testing | 3 | 90% |
| 11 | Percentage of patients with record of blood pressure | 3 | 90% |
| 12 | Percentage of patients with BP ≤148/85 mmHg | 17 | 55% |
| 13 | Percentage of patients with microalbuminuria testing (excluding those with proteinuria) | 3 | 90% |
| 14 | Percentage of patients with record of serum creatinine | 3 | 90% |
| 15 | Percentage of patients with microalbuminuria on ACEI/A2RA | 3 | 70% |
| 16 | Percentage of patients with record of total cholesterol | 3 | 90% |
| 17 | Percentage of these patients whose last measured  total cholesterol was <5 | 6 | 60% |
| 18 | Percentage of patients with influenza immunisation in previous winter | 3 | 85% |

* See also reference 4.
[†] Except where stated, all subsequent measures are the percentage of patients with known diabetes who have met the criterion *in the previous 15 months*.

### 10.4 What are the most common reasons for failing to achieve a reasonable standard in a process of care audit?

Each practice is individual and the reasons for failing to achieve appropriate standards can be diverse. Some common ones are:

- inadequate identification of patients with diabetes, a vital first step
- poor recall or clerical procedures
- inadequate documentation of what is actually already being done
- delegation of procedures to those inadequately trained for the role
- limited recognition of the clinical importance of the procedure.

### 10.5 In which aspects of care can outcome audits be undertaken?

True outcomes occur after many years, and events such as development of proliferative retinopathy should be infrequent in small practices. Information and audit of these indicators is best undertaken at a population (district, regional or national) level. Surrogate outcome indicators are therefore often used to provide earlier, more local information (*Table 10.3*). In diabetes, this includes HbA1c for glycaemic control, as long-term studies such as the UKPDS and DCCT have shown a positive correlation between HbA1c levels and the incidence of microvascular complications (*see Ch. 2*).

Some specialist units regularly calculate mean HbA1c for their patients but this often shows little change from year to year, and does not necessarily lead to significant improvements. It is preferable to calculate the percentage of patients achieving target levels of HbA1c or, better still, produce a

**TABLE 10.3  Some suggested outcome indicators for diabetes care***

|  | Surrogate | Outcome indicator and measures |
| --- | --- | --- |
| Glycaemic control | HbA1c | Incidence of microvascular complications |
| Microvascular disease | Given level of retinopathy | Cases requiring laser therapy for retinopathy |
|  | Given level of proteinuria | Cases requiring renal replacement therapy |
| Macrovascular disease | Blood pressure Cholesterol | Incidence of stroke, myocardial infarction, sudden death |
|  | Cardiovascular risk | Angioplasty rates for coronary, carotid and femoral occlusions |

* These outcomes would only be frequent enough for meaningful analysis in a large group practice or co-operative study.

frequency distribution. The proportion of poorly controlled patients (e.g. HbA1c >10%) can be reviewed annually. This can be disappointing as the patients in this group may be the most difficult to help, while the 'successes' have been discharged! This is better done in primary care.

Another way is to look at a particular patient group and review their standard of care. In one county-wide audit, all the patients treated with diet alone were identified and the records of those with HbA1c >6.5% were audited 12 months later; focusing on this particular group led to an improvement in control and this number was significantly reduced. The audit targeted a group where improving control was relatively straightforward, and highlighted the need to start oral hypoglycaemic agents sooner. A similar exercise with hypertension led to a marked increase in the proportion achieving targets.

For complications or risk factors for example, a small audit might check that everyone with microalbuminuria or proteinuria is treated with an angiotensin converting enzyme (ACE) inhibitor or angiotensin 2 (A2) blocker, or, alternatively, that those with macrovascular disease or at high risk are being treated with aspirin. An assessment of patients on lipid-lowering treatment could measure the proportion reaching target cholesterol or cardiovascular risk levels.

In the UK, national clinical audit is being started in 2004 (*see www.nhsia.nhs/uk/ncasp*).

---

### 10.6 How do you assess patient satisfaction with diabetes care?

The most straightforward way is to ask patients to complete a questionnaire! But for optimal feedback, this needs to be carefully designed. Most hospital clinical governance/quality control departments have considerable experience in this area and are happy to provide advice. It is best to tackle a limited area of care rather than the whole process of diabetes care in one go.

For more informal feedback, small focus discussion groups can be valuable. Patients often have a different perspective from the professionals and frequently suggest minor changes, which can make a dramatic difference to the system. For example, one group of patients asked to have a copy of their laboratory results prior to the consultation, so that they could prepare questions. This led to more interactive consultations and patients were happier as they had a better understanding of the results and their treatment goals.

---

### 10.7 Should high-quality diabetes care be rewarded?

Job satisfaction and improvement in the daily lives and prognosis for patients should be the reward that most health care professionals seek. However, in the UK the government has recognised that primary care is run as a business and financial incentives are a powerful tool in improving care.

This is the thinking behind the challenging specific targets for diabetes care with a points system linked to payment for a range of key audit targets (*see Table 10.2*).

## HOW MUCH DIABETES TO EXPECT IN A PRACTICE

### 10.8 How many people with diabetes are there in the average solo or group general practice?

This will vary depending upon the age distribution, ethnic mix and obesity levels in the population covered by the practice. Above-average prevalence will be found with high proportions of older patients, large populations of non-Europeans and with low socio-economic status. Lower prevalences would be expected in younger, affluent areas with mainly Europeans.

Examples of the approximate expected prevalence of known diabetes for a single-handed GP with 2000 patients and a group practice with a total of 15 000 patients (all ages, including the expected number with type 1 diabetes) are shown in *Table 10.4*.

| TABLE 10.4 Approximate prevalence of known diabetes in single-handed and group practices | | |
|---|---|---|
| | 2000 single-handed practice | 15 000 group practice |
| **UK** | | |
| Type 2 diabetes | 40–60 | 300–450 |
| Type 1 diabetes | 4–12 | 25–50 |
| **Australia/NZ/UK areas with high non-European populations** | | |
| Type 2 diabetes | 60–120 | 450–900 |
| Type 1 diabetes | 4–12 | 25–50 |

Generally there are as many cases of undiagnosed diabetes as there are with known diabetes, unless systematic screening has previously occurred. Additionally there will be many cases of impaired glucose tolerance (IGT) and impaired fasting glucose (IFG), and yet more still of the 'metabolic syndrome'.

A simple comparison of apparent diabetes prevalence in a practice, compared with other national and especially local figures, may be a useful initial audit measure.

### 10.9 What about diabetes registers?

High-quality diabetes care is virtually, if not totally, impossible without an accurate, up-to-date list of people with known diabetes; these are well developed in many practices and districts. This forms the 'denominator' from which the number of processes can be assessed for completeness; it also gives an idea of diabetes prevalence. Take for example two practices near each other of similar sizes and serving similar populations:

■ *Practice A*: 8300 patients, 210 patients on register, 166 with eyescreen in last year, 79% of register screened.
■ *Practice B*: 8500 patients, 154 patients on register, 139 with eyescreen in last year, 90% of register screened.

At first sight, Practice B may appear better at performing eye screening with 90% (139/154) of patients screened while Practice A has only performed 79%. However the prevalence in Practice A is 2.5% while that in Practice B is apparently 1.8%. If the populations are really similar in age, sex, ethnicity and social distribution, Practice B may have a less complete register accounting for the difference. In that case perhaps 50 or more patients have had no systematic care!

Possible sources of data to set up or improve a register include the following (though some may involve privacy issues):[5,6]

■ A manual or computer search of the practice database
■ A search of prescriptions for insulin, metformin, sulphonylureas, monitoring strips, etc.
■ A listing of practice patients from local secondary care services (e.g. retinal photography lists, district diabetes registers)
■ Printouts of patient lists from local pathology laboratories (e.g. for HbA1c/microalbumin)
■ Liaison with local pharmacies on dispensed prescriptions (e.g. for urine/blood testing strips).

### 10.10 What needs to be done to keep the diabetes register accurate?

Once a register has been established, a careful system is needed to maintain its accuracy using the additions/deletions outlined in *Box 10.1*.

Whilst this may seem obvious, the actual mechanisms and person responsible for making the changes must be carefully defined. For example, new cases may be diagnosed through many mechanisms, different members of the practice or other external health service activity. Is the mechanism for adding them robust enough to pick up all these sources?

A regular (at least annual) check of the register against a prescription search and the hospital/secondary services patient register is imperative to maintain accuracy.

---

### BOX 10.1  Additions/deletions to a practice diabetes register

■ Additions:
  — newly diagnosed people with diabetes
  — established diabetic patients registering for the first time with the practice
■ Deletions
  — people with diabetes who have died
  — people with diabetes who have moved away from the practice
  — some patients with gestational diabetes following pregnancy
  — patients with transient diabetes related to steroid use

---

## SPECIALIST SERVICES AND OTHER IMPORTANT COLLABORATORS

### 10.11 What specialist services should be available?

An adult diabetes service should be available without unreasonable waiting lists and have access to most, if not all, of the services outlined in *Box 10.2*.

The ease of access will vary, but optimally all the specialists mentioned will have particular expertise and interest in diabetes.

---

### 10.12 Are there any standard referral and access criteria for specialist services?

Whilst there will be understandable regional and national variation in these recommendations, there is general agreement about the need for certain groups of patients to be referred including:

■ patients with diabetic ketoacidosis or hyperosmolar non-ketotic coma
■ all children and teenagers with diabetes
■ people with newly diagnosed type 1 diabetes
■ pregnant women with diabetes, ideally pre-conception, for pre-pregnancy counselling
■ all diabetic patients with sight-threatening retinopathy

---

### BOX 10.2  Specialist services in adult diabetes care

■ Diabetes nurse specialists/educators
■ Specialist physicians
■ Dietitians
■ Podiatrists
■ Retinal photography or equivalent service
■ Ophthalmologists
■ Obstetricians
■ Nephrologists
■ Cardiologists
■ Vascular surgeons
■ Psychologists

- all diabetic patients with nephropathy
- all diabetic patients with foot ulcers.

There will be local variation in relation to problems with glycaemic control, insulin treatment, macrovascular complications and other problems.

Practices and individuals vary greatly in their knowledge of diabetes, interest, available time and resources. Best quality arises when primary and secondary care provide *complementary* care, but consistent excessive waiting times are often, if not usually, due to inadequate service provision or funding.

### 10.13 What is an LDSAG or LIT?

LDSAG stands for the local diabetes service advisory group, LIT for local implementation team. In an attempt to improve care nationally, Diabetes UK recommended that each district establish an LDSAG, to review diabetes services and promote high-quality care addressing areas of deficiency by lobbying local health authorities and service providers. Most groups comprise representation from all disciplines involved in diabetes care (both primary and secondary) and include patient representatives.

Since publication of the NSFs,[1,2] the LIT has taken over from the LDSAG. The groups are similar except that the LIT is chaired and organised by the local primary care trust whereas the LDSAGs were often organised with secondary care taking the lead role.

### 10.14 What is the role of national and local diabetes lay associations?

National diabetes societies (e.g. Diabetes UK, Diabetes Australia, Diabetes New Zealand) have been at the forefront of improvements in diabetes care for decades. Without their pressure, services would be far less satisfactory than they are today. All provide advocacy (e.g. political pressure on governments and health departments), as well as information and support to individuals with diabetes and to health professionals caring for diabetes. They have led the way in providing educational and other material, often in many languages. Many injustices experienced by those with diabetes (e.g. employment bans, driving restrictions, sport limitations) have been challenged through the societies' publicity and, on occasion, legal action through the courts. Most also have local branches and/or patient support groups (*see Appendix 3*).

### 10.15 Do guidelines help?

Guidelines should, and usually do, represent the best evidence-based summary of current practice. They do, however, tend to be lengthy and hard work to read – they also become out-of-date very quickly as new studies are published! Fortunately, they often contain a summary of the main points or are produced in a concise form for everyday use. Increasingly, they are available on the Internet, allowing easy access and identification through search engines. Recent relevant guidelines and similar material are detailed in Appendix 3.[7–11]

## CONTINUING CARE

### 10.16 What is the point of an annual review for people with diabetes?

A good analogy for patients is the MoT (Ministry of Transport) or WoF (Warrant of Fitness) test for cars – preventive maintenance rather than repair of breakdowns. It is perhaps strange that care for cars is mandatory, but that for people with diabetes optional!

Ideally, all the goals summarised above should be covered in the annual review, but time and other limits may mean it has to be split over several visits. The main clinical aim is to screen for the long-term complications, and review the risk factors for macrovascular disease.

It is essential to have a clear structure for this process to make sure it is complete. Activities can be shared between the nurse and doctor, and it is useful to have a clerical staff member prepare the records prior to the visit, checking that all necessary information is available. In the complicated patient, it may be better to undertake aspects of education and glycaemic control adjustment at an alternative visit. As can be seen from *Box 10.3*, this is not a quick 10-minute exercise!

---

**BOX 10.3  Suggested protocol for annual review**

1. Laboratory blood tests taken 1–2 weeks before visit to ensure the results are available for the consultation:
   — fasting plasma glucose
   — HbA1c
   — fasting lipid profile: total cholesterol, triglyceride, HDL and LDL cholesterol and total cholesterol:HDL ratio
   — serum creatinine
   — urine for microalbuminuria screen
   — other drug-specific needs (e.g. LFTs if thiazolidinedione or statins are being used or considered, and possibly creatine phosphokinase if statins are being used)
2. Request patient to bring:
   — urine sample: test for protein using dipstick
   — home blood glucose monitoring records
   — current medication or a complete up-to-date list

**BOX 10.3 (*Cont'd*) Suggested protocol for annual review**

3. Interview topics:
   — general health problems, including any 'events' in past year (e.g. laser-treated retinopathy or cataract, myocardial infarction, foot ulcer)
   — review of glycaemic control
   — patient's concerns: allow time for this, prompting if needed (e.g. hypos, impotence)

4. Examination:
   — weight (and height if not already recorded): calculate BMI $(kg/m^2)$
   — consider waist circumference, especially if metabolic syndrome present
   — blood pressure
   — feet: general examination, peripheral pulses and sensation using monofilament test fibres or cotton wool (*see Fig. 17.2*)
   — distant visual acuity on Snellen chart, dilated pupils for retinal photography or fundoscopy (if not performed elsewhere)
   — injection sites if on insulin
   — any sites specifically suggested by history/clinical concerns

5. Complication screening (explain results to patient):
   — retinopathy: photograph or fundoscopy findings
   — nephropathy: urine for microalbuminuria, serum creatinine, blood pressure
   — neuropathy: sensation testing, peripheral pulses

6. Risk factors for macrovascular disease and consider treatment:
   — smoking and exercise
   — blood pressure: need for intervention or adjustment of treatment
   — lipid profile and cardiovascular risk score (UKPDS or Framingham, *see Qs 13.13–13.15*): need for treatment or adjustment
   — need for low-dose aspirin

7. Educational update

8. Document findings and action in patient's notes and the patient-held record if any

9. Conclusions linking general health, glycaemic control, complication risk or management and macrovascular disease risk management

10. Arrange appropriate follow-up and make any necessary referrals/arrangements

## 10.17 Do patients with diabetes need to be seen more than once per year?

The UKPDS showed that type 2 diabetes results in gradual worsening of glycaemic control, even under research conditions with 3-monthly visits. The rate of deterioration varies between individuals, reflecting the underlying declining pancreatic beta-cell function. During a 12-month period, glycaemic control may worsen significantly without the patient being aware, especially if home monitoring is infrequent. Thus the maximum interval between visits to assess glycaemic control should probably be 6 months, or less if control is deteriorating and/or and medication needs adjustment.

Uncomplicated patients may need only 6-monthly review, but the more complex the patient and the greater the medication, the more often they need to be seen. There are no hard and fast rules (nor is there an evidence-based answer), but many people probably need input *at least* every 3 months.

There is evidence that some high-risk patients (e.g. with microalbuminuria or clinical nephropathy) actually have optimal outcomes with 3-monthly specialist follow-up.[12] Few specialist units can currently provide this.

## 10.18 What should be done at these intervening visits?

The patient's outstanding problems (clinical and psychosocial) and unmet targets will drive this. Clinically, glycaemic control, BP and dyslipidaemia are the commonest issues and there is a continuing need to listen to and educate the patient. It is helpful to reassess the last annual review results to see what the outstanding issues are. A structured consultation is ideal, but flexibility to adapt to the patient's agenda is important. It is sensible to compile a checklist for the routine follow-up visit at the end of the annual review (*Box 10.4*).

---

### BOX 10.4  Suggested protocol for a routine visit

- Laboratory tests 1–2 weeks before visit: fasting glucose and HbA1c, plus other tests indicated after or between annual reviews
- Listen to the patient's main concerns
- Weight and any changes from last visit
- Review general health including issues outside diabetes
- Review home monitoring results and HbA1c
- Review equipment: meter, insulin injection devices if used
- Deal with outstanding issues (e.g. hypertension control, smoking, foot care)
- Adjust medication for diabetes and other problems
- Review complication and risk factor management if required
- Educate and motivate
- Decide when next follow-up needed and what for

---

## 10.19 Are there special issues in dealing with diabetes in the elderly?

Increasing longevity and population changes make this a major issue, which has not received enough attention. Recent reports from the USA[13] and Australia1[4] have examined the issues in detail and make a number of recommendations:

■ Fit, elderly people should be reviewed similarly and treated along similar lines to younger people with diabetes.
■ The dangers of hypoglycaemia may require upward adjustment of targets for glycaemic control.
■ A reasonable treatment target for blood pressure is 140/90 mmHg.
■ Cognitive function should be assessed by mini-mental state examination (MMSE) as there is evidence of cognitive impairment with diabetes.
■ The frail elderly may require modification of assessments and targets.

Specific issues raised by the American group were:

■ Polypharmacy, requiring careful review, simplification where possible and clear education of patient and/or carer
■ An increased incidence of depression
■ An increased risk of falls and urinary incontinence
■ An increased incidence of persistent pain, especially from peripheral neuropathy.

---

**PQ** PATIENT QUESTIONS

### 10.20 What care should people with diabetes expect?

Diabetes UK, the patient organisation, produces an excellent leaflet for patients about the diabetes care they should expect.[15] This information is also available on their website (*www.diabetes.org.uk/infocentre*). For example, they advise that, once your diabetes is reasonably controlled, you should:

■ have access to your diabetes care team at least once a year – in this session, take the opportunity to discuss how your diabetes affects you as well as your diabetes control
■ be able to contact any member of your diabetes care team for specialist advice, in person or by telephone
■ have further education sessions when you are ready for them
■ have a formal medical review once a year with a doctor experienced in diabetes.

There is a wealth of other relevant information on the website, too extensive to reference individually.

PATIENT QUESTIONS

### 10.21  What qualifications do health care professionals need to look after people with diabetes?

■ Consultants or specialists in diabetes have completed higher medical training and, in most countries, are included in a specialist register held by the General Medical Council or similar body.

■ Diabetes nurse specialists/educators, dietitians and podiatrists will have undertaken further training and, often, specialist courses to work in the area of diabetes.

Increasingly, health care professionals in primary care are taking courses to train beyond the basics in diabetes care, and there are extensive training and update courses available.

# Issues of daily life with diabetes

## ALTERNATIVE TREATMENTS

### PQ PATIENT QUESTIONS

Diabetes has a major impact on everyday life, and the stresses and activities of daily life have an impact on diabetes. The well-adapted patient accepts and understands these interactions, making appropriate compromises and monitoring the effects. This chapter examines some of these issues and links closely with Chapter 4 covering dietary topics, exercise, smoking and alcohol.

## MONITORING GLYCAEMIC CONTROL

### 11.1 Why, how and when should patients monitor their diabetes?

Everyone with diabetes has their personal version, which they have to live with every day. Successful management depends on acceptance of the condition and learning to take control. Asking the patient to monitor their own diabetes is the first step in this. Once confidence develops, most will experiment with diet to see the effects of eating both the right and wrong types of food, and of exercise and stress on their control.

Testing urine for glucose with a dipstick, or checking a fingerprick capillary glucose sample with increasingly small meters, are the options for day-to-day monitoring. Many patients are automatically taught home blood glucose monitoring (HBGM), some countries have now virtually withdrawn urine-testing materials.

### 11.2 How good is the evidence on the value of blood glucose self-testing?

There is no evidence that blood glucose self-testing is superior to urine testing for glycaemic control: a randomised controlled trial in people with newly diagnosed diabetes showed no significant difference at 6 months.[1] Urine testing is significantly cheaper and easier. With a normal renal threshold for glucose of approximately 10 mmol/l, a well-controlled patient should find all their urine tests are negative. The renal threshold for glucose varies and a few people have a lower renal threshold, with glycosuria occurring at normal blood glucose (BG) levels. Conversely, some have a higher renal threshold with glycosuria not occurring until BG exceeds 12–15 mmol/l – this is not uncommon amongst the elderly. For patients using urine testing, it is important to compare the results with laboratory plasma glucose (PG) values and HbA1c to ensure they do not have an abnormal renal threshold and that the method is appropriately sensitive. Urine testing obviously cannot detect hypoglycaemia.

> Home BG monitoring is easy with modern meters, which can give a result in 5–20 seconds with a tiny volume of blood – many also have a memory facility. Patients like to see the effect of food or exercise on their BG but many become frustrated when they find varying results with no clear reason. To gain maximum benefit from blood testing, patients should be able to adjust not only their diet but also their medication. At present it is unusual for tablet-treated patients to be taught this.

### 11.3 When exactly should patients undertake blood glucose testing?

The limited evidence for the value of capillary BG testing alone has already been discussed (*see Q. 7.1*); there have been no trials to date about optimal times for testing. A sensible (but not evidence-based) approach is to look at the reasons for testing which include:

- informing the patient of how well their diabetes is being controlled, and whether any changes in treatment are needed
- providing information to other medical advisors for the same reasons
- detecting imminent hypoglycaemia if the patient is at risk
- helping with diabetes management during periods of instability due to exercise, changes in food intake, stress or illness.

Thus timing and frequency of testing will vary with the clinical situation as outlined in *Box 11.1* and *Table 11.1*.

### 11.4 Are there any downsides to self-testing?

 Sore fingers are the obvious ones! It is less painful to test on the side of the finger than on the pulp. There are also issues of over-anxiety and frequent adjustment of insulin doses that can lead to unstable control (*see Q. 11.3*), often due to excessive or too frequent additional insulin doses. Others who perform self-testing as a routine and neither use the results to inform themselves nor their carers are probably wasting their own time as well as expensive resources – testing strips cost the country as much as tablets and insulin combined!

### 11.5 Can alternative sites to the fingers be used to test?

Yes, but with some limitations. Some meters are now designed to work on the forearm. In general, studies show good correlations between these and finger capillary glucose levels for stable BG concentrations (e.g. fasting and pre-prandial ones), less good for hypoglycaemic and post-prandial samples. Fingerprick capillary circulation is usually brisk and reflects prevailing BG levels. Other alternate sites may have a more sluggish circulation especially if the air temperature is low. This means the *capillary blood* glucose may not

---

**BOX 11.1 Timing and frequency of blood glucose self-testing**

■ Patient on diet alone or OHAs:
— may monitor using urine testing rather than BG testing
— might undertake a daily urine test or perhaps two or three tests on 2 days per week, varying the timing between before and after meals
— should aim for all urine tests to be negative
— might test before and 1.5–2 hours after breakfast and/or the main meal to show roughly 'minimum' and 'maximum' values if BG testing is used
■ Patients on insulin, with or without OHAs:
— should ideally undertake BG testing
— should test before and 1.5–2 hours after breakfast and the main meal to show roughly 'minimum' and 'maximum' values
— should undertake daily BG testing but varying the times during the day
— should do occasional tests *at times of hypoglycaemia risk* (e.g. fasting, pre-lunch, pre-dinner, after exercise)
— may need to increase testing for occupational reasons or if frequent hypoglycaemia is a problem
— may undertake once-daily testing at variable times, if found to be sufficient
■ Patients on more complex insulin regimens, including those with type 1 diabetes:
— may undertake once-daily testing at variable times, if found to be sufficient
— may need more frequent testing to detect hypoglycaemia and post-prandial hyperglycaemia
— may need to test more often if variable lifestyle, varying eating patterns and exercise necessitate frequent insulin dose adjustment
— should not usually exceed about four tests per day, except for pregnancy and those with hypoglycaemic unawareness or during unstable periods.
— need to be aware that too many tests can lead to anxiety and swinging BG levels, often due to frequent inappropriate self-adjustment of insulin, and sometimes diet as well

---

be an absolutely accurate reflection of *venous plasma* glucose. Patients must therefore be aware of this when using such a method. It is particularly important to use fingerprick testing if hypoglycaemia is suspected, as alternate site testing can have a 10–15-minute lag in reflecting this.

**TABLE 11.1 Example of blood testing results**

| Day | Date | Breakfast Before | Breakfast After | Lunch Before | Lunch After | Dinner Before | Dinner After | Bedtime | Overnight | Comment |
|---|---|---|---|---|---|---|---|---|---|---|
| **Patient with type 2 diabetes on metformin and sulphonylurea** | | | | | | | | | | |
| Mon | 7.7.03 | | | | | | | | | |
| Tues | 8.7.03 | | | | | | | | | |
| Wed | 9.7.03 | 8.4 | | | | | 9.8 | | | |
| Thurs | 10.7.03 | | | | | | | | | |
| Fri | 11.7.03 | | | | | | | | | |
| Sat | 12.7.03 | | | | | | | | | |
| Sun | 13.7.03 | 7.3 | | | 13.2 | | | | | Big family lunch |

Comments: *Adequate testing pattern that suggests inadequate glycaemic control.*

| Day | Date | Breakfast Before | Breakfast After | Lunch Before | Lunch After | Dinner Before | Dinner After | Bedtime | Overnight | Comment |
|---|---|---|---|---|---|---|---|---|---|---|
| **Patient on nocturnal insulin and metformin** | | | | | | | | | | |
| Mon | 11.8.03 | 5.2 | | | | | | | | |
| Tues | 12.8.03 | | | | 9.2 | | 11.4 | | | |
| Wed | 13.8.03 | 5.5 | | | | | | | | |
| Thurs | 14.8.03 | | | 4.2 | | | | 12.1 | | Gardening ++ all morning |
| Fri | 15.8.03 | | 9.5 | | | | | | | |
| Sat | 16.8.03 | 6.9 | | | | 8.8 | | | | Got up late |
| Sun | 17.8.03 | | | | | | | | | Walk in evening |

Comments: *Good testing pattern; good overnight control; less good late afternoon/evening. Note effect of gardening.*

| Day | Date | Breakfast Before | Breakfast After | Lunch Before | Lunch After | Dinner Before | Dinner After | Bedtime | Overnight | Comment |
|---|---|---|---|---|---|---|---|---|---|---|
| **Active patient with type 1 diabetes on Actrapid and protophane regimen** | | | | | | | | | | |
| Mon | 18.8.03 | 7.6 | | 3.6 | | | | 7.8 | | Late for lunch |
| Tues | 19.8.03 | 8.3 | | | | 7.0 | | | | Run in evening |
| Wed | 20.8.03 | 3.9 | 11.5 | | 10.1 | | 10.7 | | | |
| Thurs | 21.8.03 | | 15.1 | | | 8.6 | | | 5.6 | Run in evening |
| Fri | 22.8.03 | 4.4 | | | 5.2 | | | 12.3 | | Evening meal out |
| Sat | 23.8.03 | 10.1 | | | | 10.3 | | | | } Wet weather, lazy weekend |
| Sun | 24.8.03 | 8.6 | | 5.3 | | 12.2 | | | | } |

Comments: *Intelligent use of testing: note effects of late lunch, exercise and 'lazy weekend'. Also high post-prandial glucoses; might benefit from switch to NovoRapid. May need lower bedtime protophane dose after running, and ? higher dose otherwise.*

### 11.6 How about these clever devices that read through the skin?

Devices such as the 'Glucowatch' or 'MiniMed sensor' have been devised to read interstitial fluid glucose. The good news is that they mirror BG reasonably accurately though there may be a small delay; less good is the cumbersome technology and that they must be calibrated against a standard method (fingerprick blood test) and require new electrodes every 12 hours or 2–3 days. They are additionally very expensive.

They have considerable value in showing patterns of BG over 12 hours or 24–48-hour periods (depending on the sensor type), which may be valuable as a diagnostic tool. They often show periods of unrecognised hypoglycaemia, especially overnight, that are not detected by conventional monitoring – and thus prompt treatment changes.

The technology is not yet sufficiently robust or affordable for patients to use frequently or to form the basis of 'closing the loop' with an insulin pump to produce an 'artificial pancreas'.

## PSYCHOLOGICAL ISSUES, DEPRESSION AND STRESS

### 11.7 What are the common psychological problems associated with the diagnosis of diabetes?

This has been an under-recognized area in specialist care, though general practice has been only too aware of it![2] Some specialist centres have a clinical psychologist with experience in diabetes: commonly identified problems are outlined in *Box 11.2*

Several problems are commoner in type 1 diabetes. Fear of hypoglycaemia and lack of acceptance of the need for insulin are common presenting complaints, but often have roots long before the presentation of diabetes.

As well as this, it is essential to be aware of the psychological model of readiness for change in behaviour (*see Appendix 1*).

---

**BOX 11.2 Psychological problems commonly associated with the diagnosis of diabetes**

- Depression/grief
- Anxiety, especially in the early years
- Non-acceptance of diabetes
- Difficulty in adjustment to diabetes
- Issues of eating, body image, weight management (especially in type 1 diabetes)
- Interpersonal problems
- Stress
- Sexual dysfunction

---

### 11.8 How common is depression in type 2 diabetes?

> Depression is significantly more common than in the general population.[3–5] Many studies have shown this for patients with both type 2 and type 1 diabetes, though it is not clear whether this is more so with diabetes than for other long-term disorders (e.g. severe asthma or arthritis).
>
> What is clear is that depression frequently manifests itself in terms of poor control; treatment then directed at tablet or insulin modification is unlikely to be effective. Standard tools of assessment are useful, but the greatest need is for a low threshold of suspicion, especially when these patients are familiar to their caring team.
>
> There are some treatment differences: specific serotonin reuptake inhibitors (SSRIs) are the drugs of choice rather than tricyclic antidepressants. The latter can lead to significant problems with postural hypotension.

## THE EFFECT OF DIABETES ON OTHER CONDITIONS

---

### 11.9 What about the effect of intercurrent illness on diabetes?

This is a vitally important question and is dealt with in detail in Chapter 9.

---

### 11.10 Can and should patients with diabetes have their usual vaccinations? Are any special ones needed?

In general, no changes to the usual recommendations are necessary,[6] though some experts would avoid giving these while diabetes is poorly controlled.

Diabetes is usually included in the list of patients recommended for annual influenza immunisation – this now part of the contract performance indicators (*see Table 10.2*). There is limited evidence to support this recommendation, based on the belief that people with diabetes are more susceptible to infections, which is probably only true if diabetes control is poor. However, influenza is likely to lead to significant deterioration in glucose control, which could be serious in frail or poorly controlled patients; certainly hospital admissions tend to be prolonged. For younger, well-controlled patients entirely free of complications, annual influenza vaccine is not essential but is desirable.

Pneumococcal vaccine is advocated by some experts and many guidelines on the basis of a significantly increased risk of pneumococcal disease; this has not become a widespread practice and the cost:benefit ratio is not clear.

### 11.11 Do insulin and diabetic drugs interact or give problems with any other drugs?

There is a long list of potential interactions in the BNF but few of these are significant or common enough to be relevant. The obvious exception is steroids which seriously affect glycaemic control when used in doses above an equivalent of prednisolone 5–7 mg/day (*see Q. 9.6*). Otherwise for insulin the answer really is no serious interactions.

Though there are a number of listed interactions for oral hypoglycaemic agents (OHAs) and commonly used drugs, only the following are significant enough to be mentioned; practical problems are rare in practice:

- Sulphonylurea effects possibly increased by sulphonamides, ciprofloxacin, warfarin, antifungals
- Warfarin: effect enhanced by fibrates.

### 11.12 Are there any other precautions that people with diabetes should take?

Patients on insulin, and those on sulphonylureas who are prone to hypoglycaemia, are usually advised to have a MedicAlert bracelet or necklace (*see Appendix 3*); this will alert anyone who finds the patient unconscious. A cheaper (but less satisfactory) solution is an identity card kept in the purse or wallet – pharmaceutical companies often supply these. It is additionally wise to make sure that close friends and colleagues are aware of a patient's diabetes if there is any chance of hypoglycaemia.

## EMPLOYMENT AND DRIVING

### 11.13 What jobs will not be permitted for someone with diabetes?

The majority of restrictions on occupations for people with diabetes relate to the risk of hypoglycaemia and treatment employed (insulin and/or sulphonylureas), rather than to the presence of diabetes itself. Thus there are a number of prohibited occupations for patients with type 1 diabetes. They will often also be barred for those with type 2 diabetes who require insulin, even though the risk of hypoglycaemia is much less. Common examples in the UK and elsewhere include:

- commercial airline, and usually recreational, pilots – also usually cabin crew
- armed forces
- police
- train drivers
- jobs requiring heavy goods vehicle (HGV) or passenger carrying vehicle (PCV) licence
- offshore work.

While some of these are absolute bans, in other countries there is an element of discretion and jobs may be permitted under strict conditions and expert medical supervision. The situation with those treated with sulphonylureas is more complex, though far fewer occupations are entirely closed.

Usually people on diet or metformin will be *allowed to continue in a career they have already embarked upon,* though any form of diabetes may be a disqualification from *entering* this occupation because of the likely use of sulphonylurea or insulin treatment at a later date. It is valuable for an individual to request an exact statement of why employment is being refused on health grounds.

Sulphonylurea drugs (and meglitinides) have a substantially lower risk of hypoglycaemia than insulin and may not involve the same restrictions. However, each country and each situation is different, and there is often considerable variation even between different public sector employers within the same country.

Several complications of diabetes can affect suitability for employment, for example impaired vision, cardiovascular disease, neuropathy and foot problems. In general these are treated in the same way as for someone without diabetes.

Patient organisations such as Diabetes UK are well informed of the current restrictions, which can and do change; they are also often extremely effective in lobbying.

### 11.14 How do I assess a patient's fitness for holding a driving licence?

In the UK, patients holding or applying for a Class 1 licence must declare their diabetes to the DVLA if insulin or tablets are used, but not if they are treated by diet (and lifestyle) alone. All those applying for a Class 2 licence (for HGV or PCV) must declare diabetes even if on diet alone. Detailed regulations are available on the DVLA website (*www.dvla.govt.uk*) (*see also Q. 7.14*).

Assuming the patient's general health is satisfactory, with no major complications (e.g. laser-treated retinopathy or cataract, which are specifically mentioned on the application form), the main issue is the risk of hypoglycaemia.[7] Excellent recognition of hypoglycaemia by the patient and appropriate action is the key. Those people with lack of awareness of hypoglycaemia should not be driving. This is fortunately substantially less in type 2 than in type 1 diabetes, the basic rules for which are outlined in *Table 11.2.*

### 11.15 What are the rules about commercial driving in type 2 diabetes?

These are complex and fairly restrictive in the UK and Europe, but more flexible and evidence based in other countries. The current UK regulations are found on the DVLA website (*www.dvla.gov.uk*) (*see also Appendix 3*).

**TABLE 11.2  Treatment of type 2 diabetes and related hypoglycaemia risk**

| Treatment | Hypoglycaemia risk |
|---|---|
| Diet alone or with metformin | No risk |
| Sulphonylurea/meglitinide (with or without metformin) | Small risk |
|  | Highest risk before meals |
| Insulin (with or without oral agents) | Higher risk of hypoglycaemia (still less than type 1) |
|  | Commoner with multiple injection regimens |
|  | Commoner with very 'tight' control |
|  | Highest risk at peak times of relevant insulins |

## 11.16 Can people who have retinopathy continue driving?

The decision depends upon the patient's distant visual acuity (VA) and the visual fields if laser photocoagulation has been undertaken. In the UK, all drivers must be able to read a car number plate at 20.5 metres which equates to a distant VA between 6/9 and 6/12 on a Snellen chart. Laser treatment for proliferative retinopathy can lead to significant restriction of visual fields and in the UK, patients must undergo a formal visual field assessment which is submitted to the DVLA; these examinations must be undertaken by an ophthalmologist or optometrist.

## CULTURAL AND LINGUISTIC ISSUES

## 11.17 What cultural issues relevant to diabetes are seen in different populations?

This is far too big a question to answer in a paragraph or two, and much of it is not specific to diabetes. There are, however, a number of particularly relevant and common issues which should briefly be mentioned:

■ *Ramadan fasting in patients on insulin or sulphonylureas*: During this period, healthy Muslim adults take no food or drink during daylight hours, with large meals before dawn and after dark. While those who are sick are excused, many people with diabetes take part. Those on insulin or sulphonylureas may need advice to reduce, re-time or alter their medication, whereas metformin doses should be taken with the actual meals. Advice needs to be individualised – a nurse educator will usually have encountered this before.

■ *Avoidance of pork insulin by Jews*: Important to remember, but no longer much of a problem.

■ *Unwillingness to acknowledge a diagnosis of diabetes as being shameful or self-inflicted*: This is common in many cultures but in most is becoming less common with increasing publicity.

■ *Reluctance to lose weight*: Older Afro-Caribbean women will usually ignore advice to lose weight as 'bigger is better' as far as their partners are concerned.

■ *Male/female health provider issues*: Several religions and cultures will not (or find very difficult to) accept examination of a woman by a male doctor or vice versa, especially when issues related to sex or other bodily functions are concerned. In diabetes this is mainly concerned with impotence and pregnancy.

■ *Entertaining*: In Pacific Islander and Maori peoples among others, generous entertaining is important – food must never run out. For the guest it is expected that all will be consumed as a mark of appreciation/respect. The resultant problem in weight control is obvious!

■ *Understanding of chronic diseases*: Many cultures lack true appreciation of any chronic 'incurable' condition, the only understanding being of acute illness. This leads to intermittent adherence, often only taking treatment when people feel ill.

■ *Prioritisation of health*: This isn't really a cultural issue, but many patients will do without their medication if money is short, preferring it to go to food, clothing or education of the family, especially the children. This will rarely be admitted.

■ *Language*: Adequate interpreter availability is important if real understanding and education are to be achieved. This may need to be a careful balance between involvement of the patient's family, who certainly need to know much of the dietary and self-care information, and the privacy of the patient where more personal issues are being discussed. The NHS has phone translation services for many languages.

### 11.18 How does economic and social status affect diabetes?

Type 1 diabetes has a similar incidence and prevalence across social and economic classes but this is very different in type 2 diabetes which has its highest prevalence in the lowest socio-economic classes. This is largely due to the relationship with obesity, which increases in incidence across the social classes, being most common in manual workers.

Complications of diabetes and cardiovascular disease are more common in the most deprived patients. This probably is due to a combination of a long period of undiagnosed diabetes, failure to achieve adequate glycaemic control after diagnosis and poor uptake of screening and treatment for complications. Lifestyle issues of poor diet, inadequate exercise and high smoking rates contribute to poorer outcome but represent real challenges to health care professionals trying to treat this group. Patients trying to deal with major social problems are unlikely to be responsive to health care messages. Additionally healthy eating is more expensive than unhealthy eating; looking after the children may take priority. Maintaining regular contact with the patient may be the most important aim in these situations.

There is recent encouraging data from Salford that socio-economic deprivation does not preclude high-quality diabetes care.[8]

## ALTERNATIVE TREATMENTS

### 11.19 Are vitamin and mineral supplements necessary or helpful?

There is no good evidence for any systematic benefit for supplements, and most healthy diets already include nutritionally adequate amounts. The Heart Protection Study included a vitamin preparation (vitamins C and E plus beta-carotene) as one treatment arm and there was no benefit in reducing cardiovascular disease in either diabetic or non-diabetic groups. Numerous vitamins and minerals have been proposed as preventing type 2 diabetes and reducing BG in patients with diabetes, but there are as yet no conclusive studies to support these claims.[9,10] Some positive but inconclusive studies have been reported for chromium and vanadium supplements.

While conventional vitamin supplements in recommended doses do not appear to cause harm, many patients exceed these doses on the basis that 'if one is good, four must be better'! A detailed history of all medication, including 'over-the-counter', 'dietary' and 'herbal' is worthwhile.

### 11.20 What about herbal treatments to control or prevent diabetes?

A recent review[10] found insufficient evidence of systematic benefit for any firm recommendations about herbal treatments though many studies have been positive to varying degrees – those felt to warrant formal study were *Coccinia indica*, American ginseng, *Gymnema sylvestre*, *Aloe vera*, *Momordica charantia* and nopal. Some traditional remedies for diabetes have been found to have some hypoglycaemic actions in animal models of diabetes. However, several studies have shown that large proportions of populations consume these remedies on a regular basis, often at considerable expense.

There are some problems: Chinese 'herbs' in particular need to be watched: one recent instance found the traditional Chinese remedy included substantial amounts of glibenclamide – up to 10 mg/day in standard dose!

The Australian *MIMS* guide includes a useful list of interactions between herbal and conventional medications.

**PATIENT QUESTIONS**

### 11.21 Do I need to tell my employer that I have diabetes?

It is illegal in the UK and other countries to discriminate against people with diabetes for employment except for specified occupations such as the airline industry (*see Q. 11.13*). Honesty and full disclosure are, however, essential when completing any job application form with health questions, as it forms part of a legal contract. Obviously, if the occupation could pose risks in someone liable to hypoglycaemia (e.g. machinery work), then disclosure is imperative for everyone's protection. If diabetes is well controlled, then it can be declared as 'well-controlled type 2 diabetes'. Diabetes UK and other national bodies have excellent publications on this and similar areas, and will offer phone advice to members (*see Appendix 3*).

### 11.22 Can stress affect my glucose control?

Acute stress, physical or mental, certainly increases BG levels in the short term in many patients, especially in type 1 diabetes, but also in those with type 2 diabetes. This is often apparent from a patient's own diaries. It is also clear that longer-term stress may have substantial and significant effects – one study of a stress management intervention produced a mean reduction in HbA1c of 0.5% over 12 months, with levels in some of the participants dropping by over 1%, implying a major effect in many patients.[4]

### 11.23 Does diabetes affect foreign travel in any way?

Diabetes need not limit foreign travel, unless complications render it unwise (e.g. going up the Amazon when near end-stage renal failure or with active foot disease). However, there are a number of issues that need to be considered before a journey is undertaken.

**Prior to journey**

- *Long flights*: Airline meals for people with diabetes are often poor, but arrive on time. Always carry some spare carbohydrate snacks but they may need to be discarded before customs (e.g. fruit into Australia/New Zealand).
- *Hypoglycaemia avoidance*: If in doubt, run glucoses high rather than low.
- *Medical supplies – verification*: These must be labelled and in original containers, ideally with a doctor's letter or (legible!) copy of the prescription if travelling outside Western Europe – unlabelled white tablets are not appreciated by the Thai customs!
- *Medical supplies – quantities*: Take sufficient supplies for your journey in hand baggage. If staying long term, find out the availability and name of your insulin and medicines at your destination before you go.
- *Insulin*: Insulin is best kept in hand baggage as the temperature of luggage in the hold may fall below freezing. Insulin will need to be kept cool in hot countries – insulated bags are widely available.

■ *Timing of injections*: Crossing time zones can cause problems with the timing of insulin injections. Find out the details of the flight from the airline, and then get advice from your nurse educator who will be able to help with a flight plan.

**At your destination**

■ *Foods*: Be aware of the possible effects of unusual foods, especially if BGs are tightly controlled.
■ *Exercise:* Unusual patterns of exercise, both less and more, can alter your control.
■ *Hypoglycaemia*: Watch out for hypos; hot weather can cause faster insulin absorption from the skin, and reduced appetite may lead to inadequate carbohydrate intake.
■ *Illness*: Intercurrent illness (e.g. traveller's diarrhoea) may be an issue – read a travel medicine guide if you are going somewhere unusual or exotic. Good advice can be found on the Internet (*see Appendix 3*).
■ *Patient associations*: Most countries have patient diabetes associations – find out before you go.
■ *Medication*: If the supply of drugs or insulin is an issue (e.g. for emigration), talk to the company who make the product about availability, names and costs.

### 11.24 What effect does a diagnosis of type 2 diabetes have on life and health care insurance?

Life assurance policies are obtainable for most people with type 2 diabetes but with higher premiums to cover the increased risk. For some of those with complications, it may be difficult or impossible to obtain cover. Patient organisations such as Diabetes UK and other national bodies often have contacts with expert specialist brokers who can be extremely helpful – it is generally preferable to explore these options *before* putting in an application (*see Appendix 3*).

Usually, a medical report from your GP or specialist will be required, for which he will need your specific consent. It is important that you provide him with all the information he needs such as your self-testing records. The medical report asks specific questions including how good your control is, and how regularly you test and have checks.

Health care insurance is more complex. Different policies have different rules: while an initial diagnosis of diabetes may be covered, subsequent long-term care and complications are often not covered. Careful reading of policy conditions, discussion with a knowledgeable broker and assistance from patient organisations are invaluable.

### 11.25  Can I give blood?

In general, people with type 2 diabetes treated by diet and lifestyle changes alone will be able to give blood in the UK, assuming they do not have significant other medical conditions. Currently, those who are taking oral hypoglycaemic agents or insulin (thus including all those with type 1 diabetes) are not permitted to give blood, primarily because of concerns about the health of the donor. This does seem rather restrictive, as the concern is not about the transmission of the drugs.

# Reproduction and sexual function

# 12

## FERTILITY IN DIABETIC PARENTS

### 12.1 Does diabetes affect fertility and cause miscarriage?

If glycaemic control is reasonable or good, type 1 diabetes does not seem to affect fertility. However, if it is not ideal, the miscarriage rate increases, with as many as 25% of pregnancies leading to miscarriage when HbA1c is >12%. At conception and in the weeks that follow, the embryo undergoes huge developmental steps. The abnormal metabolic cellular environment associated with suboptimal glycaemic control increases the rate of abnormalities in the developing embryo (*see Case vignette 12.1*). At early stages of development many of these will be lethal, so the pregnancy aborts naturally. Other non-lethal effects are seen in the increased incidence of congenital abnormalities that occur in babies of women with diabetes.[1,2] A few are almost specific to diabetes (*see Q. 12.12*); the majority are more general.

### CASE VIGNETTE 12.1

A 22-year old woman with type 1 diabetes for 10 years, currently on twice-daily mixed insulin, sees you with her partner suspecting she may be 2 months pregnant. At clinic recently glycaemic control was poor, HbA1c 10.5%. The pregnancy is completely unplanned. She remembers that diabetes can cause problems in pregnancy, but she and her partner want to know the risks. Will the baby be all right or should they consider termination?

*Comment*

If she is pregnant and was poorly controlled at the time of conception, there is a high risk, perhaps around 10–15%, of a congenital abnormality; that said, 85–90% would not have an abnormality.

This couple need expert advice so they can make a decision about continuation of the presumed pregnancy. Apart from confirmation with a laboratory pregnancy test and an ultrasound scan to check foetal viability and give an accurate gestation date, it will be too early to detect most abnormalities. An urgent referral should be made to a joint diabetes–obstetric clinic where diabetologist, midwife and obstetrician work closely together. There then needs to be a joint assessment between GP, specialist team and the patient of how they will cope with the stress surrounding the difficult decision about whether to proceed with the pregnancy or not. In the meantime, she needs improved glycaemic control rapidly; a change to a more intensive insulin regimen with regular input from the diabetes nurse specialist will be required.

## 12.2 What is the ideal contraceptive method for a woman with diabetes?

The increased risk of congenital abnormality and the hormonal effects of pregnancy on diabetes should encourage all women with diabetes to plan their pregnancies carefully. An unplanned pregnancy can lead to major emotional and physical problems, thus contraception and the possibility of pregnancy need to be discussed with all women with diabetes in the reproductive years, particularly before they become sexually active.

The perfect contraceptive method for someone with diabetes does not exist.

- The combined oestrogen/progesterone contraceptive pill is most effective in preventing pregnancy, but synthetic oestrogen preparations are associated with a small but significant increased risk of thrombosis and arterial disease. As with a non-diabetic patient, the latter is of concern in women with diabetes who are smokers, have a family history of early arterial disease or who already have microvascular complications, especially nephropathy, making occult vascular problems more likely. It may be reasonable to choose a combined pill for the teenager or woman in her twenties when accidental pregnancy would be a disaster. When starting the pill, patients should be warned that a small increase in insulin dose is often required to overcome the oestrogenic effect of insulin antagonism. BP and lipids should also be monitored.

- The progesterone-only pill is often a better choice for the older woman with diabetes, especially those with type 2 diabetes and the metabolic syndrome, smokers or those with complications as it avoids the oestrogen problems. However this is balanced by a higher contraceptive failure rate and the need for excellent compliance to achieve optimal contraception.

- Depot parenteral progestogens make a suitable alternative if adherence is a problem, but are associated with weight gain.

- Barrier forms of contraception are valuable but require a high level of commitment to achieve a low failure rate.

- Intra-uterine devices can be used safely in diabetes provided there is no history of pelvic inflammatory disease and glycaemic control is satisfactory to minimise the small increased risk of pelvic infection.

Finally, if a woman has completed her family, permanent sterilisation of the partner is perhaps the ideal choice!

### 12.3 Does diabetes affect fertility in men?

Again, good data are few. The best evidence suggests that there are minor differences in some seminal fluid parameters, but these are not clinically significant issues unless of course the male partner has major erectile dysfunction.

### PRE-CONCEPTION

### 12.4 What is the importance of pre-conception counselling in diabetes? What areas should it cover?

Pre-conception counselling involves a thorough review of the patient's health, glycaemic control and presence of diabetic complications to minimise the risk to mother and unborn child. All women planning a pregnancy should receive pre-pregnancy counselling by an experienced clinician, as this is clearly associated with a better outcome. However, this may be because more motivated women are more likely to attend such counselling.

The areas covered need to include general pregnancy issues, a specific review of glycaemic control and the suitability of the current treatment, plus a full complication screen (*Table 12.1*).

If a patient is being treated with an angiotensin converting enzyme (ACE) inhibitor for microalbuminuria, proteinuria or hypertension, this should be stopped. If BP rises above 135/90 mmHg, alternative anti-hypertensive medications such as labetalol or methyldopa should be considered.

**TABLE 12.1  Issues to be covered at pre-conception counselling**

| General pregnancy issues | Glycaemic control | Diabetic complications |
| --- | --- | --- |
| Smoking and alcohol | HbA1c target <6.5% | Screen for retinopathy |
| Rubella status | In type 2 diabetes, stop OHAs and commence insulin. Consider need for insulin even if on diet alone | Screen for nephropathy – microalbuminuria |
| HIV status | | |
| Start folic acid | | Check BP and serum creatinine |
| Review any drugs taken, especially ACEI, or drugs for hypertension | | Screen for neuropathy |
| | In type 1 diabetes, switch to multiple injections if control inadequate | |

## PREGNANCY IN DIABETES

### 12.5 How and why does pregnancy upset diabetic control?

Pregnancy hormones have effects on glucose metabolism, generally antagonising insulin action so more insulin is required to achieve the same glycaemic control. During normal pregnancy, there is relatively little effect on plasma glucose (PG) but insulin concentrations increase dramatically between 20 and 34 weeks' gestation to counteract the effect of placental hormones. Injected insulin doses need to be similarly increased so, towards the end of pregnancy, women are taking on average about *double* their pre-pregnancy doses. Unfortunately this increase is neither predictable nor linear, so blood glucose (BG) levels need to be monitored carefully and frequently – at least four times daily including post-prandially – and dose adjustments made continuously.

In the early weeks, however, most women with type 1 diabetes find marked fluctuations in BG levels, sometimes with frequent and unexpected hypoglycaemic episodes. In many, insulin requirements fall in the first trimester. This is related to hormone effects but may also be aggravated by nausea and the patient's attempts to tightly control BG levels once she knows she is pregnant.

### 12.6 Why do some women get 'gestational diabetes'?

The formal definition of 'gestational diabetes' (GDM) is when the onset or recognition of diabetes *first occurs* in pregnancy – it thus includes patients who probably had undiagnosed type 2 diabetes before pregnancy. If the pancreas has reduced reserve, it will be unable to secrete sufficient insulin and thus PG levels rise (*see Q. 12.5*). After delivery of the baby and placenta, placental hormonal effects disappear within a few hours and *gestational* diabetes resolves. True gestational diabetes usually develops between 26 and 36 weeks' gestation but may occur earlier. Diabetes diagnosed in the first trimester is suspicious of previously unrecognised pre-existing type 2 diabetes.

The typical woman who develops GDM usually has significant risk factors, much as for type 2 diabetes:

- obese or overweight
- older
- positive family history of diabetes
- multiparity
- previous gestational diabetes
- non-European ethnicity.

GDM is seen more frequently in ethnic groups such as South and East Asian, Aboriginal, Maori, Pacific Island, American Indian and Hispanic women. Many centres now routinely screen all women at 28 weeks' gestation, especially where there are large ethnic populations. Women with GDM are at high risk of developing type 2 diabetes in the future and, after pregnancy, should be screened annually for the condition.

## 12.7 Surely type 2 diabetes in pregnancy is rare?

No longer! Until recently this was largely true in European populations, but increasing rates of obesity and delay in the age of childbirth has changed this. This is especially true where non-European populations are concerned – in these women, diagnosis of diabetes is often 7–10 years younger. Additionally, it has been recognised that many patients with apparent GDM, where the diabetes is still present post-partum, actually had previously undiagnosed type 2 diabetes.[3] Some centres now have more pregnant women with type 2 diabetes than with type 1; these women seem to have similar foetal risks to those with type 1 diabetes, but are older and more obese (*see Q. 12.6*).

## 12.8 Why are women with type 1 diabetes still considered a high-risk group in pregnancy?

Despite recent advances, pregnancy in women with type 1 diabetes is associated with increased levels of adverse outcomes, including increased perinatal mortality rate, congenital malformations, hypertensive disorders of pregnancy, polyhydramnios, macrosomia, birth trauma, operative delivery and neonatal metabolic problems (hypoglycaemia, jaundice).

The perinatal mortality rate is four to five times higher than for non-diabetic pregnancies, especially where non-specialist centres are concerned. Five times more babies are stillborn and the congenital abnormality rate remains eight to ten times higher than normal, though specialist centres may achieve better outcomes.[2,4,5]

*Table 12.2* shows why diabetes in pregnancy immediately places the woman and her baby into the high-risk category. Other groups in Scandinavia and the USA have reported better pregnancy outcomes, but even these still show significantly more problems than the background population.

Sudden unexplained intra-uterine death remains a significant anxiety in the final trimester and seems to be more common if the baby is macrosomic. For this reason many women with diabetes have been delivered 2–4 weeks before term. This leads to a high caesarean section rate and problems of prematurity for the baby. The policy in most centres is now to ensure delivery at term provided glycaemic control has been good

**TABLE 12.2 Some recent UK regional results of outcome of pregnancy in women with diabetes**

| Rate (per 1000) | Type 1 (Merseyside) | Types 1 and 2 (Northern ) | Type 1 (Norfolk) | UK background rates (non-diabetic) |
|---|---|---|---|---|
| Perinatal mortality rate | 36 | 48 | 25 | 8–9 |
| Stillbirth rate | 25 | N/A | 12 | 5.0 |
| Congenital anomaly rate | 94 | 83 | 32 | 10–21 |

N/A, not available

but, if there are concerns about macrosomia or other obstetric complications, to deliver at 38 weeks.

## 12.9 What are the likely outcomes of pregnancy in type 2 diabetes and gestational diabetes?

Recent data from one multi-ethnic population have shown that the outcomes for patients with type 2 diabetes are worse than for type 1; other studies show no difference. This applied to patients with known type 2 diabetes *and* for those newly presenting, but who remained diabetic after the pregnancy.[3] In contrast, 'true' gestational diabetes did not show any excess mortality. Unlike the pregnancies in women with type 1 diabetes, congenital abnormalities were rare as causes of perinatal mortality (*Fig. 12.1*).

Even in GDM there is clear evidence of an increased rate of macrosomia in these pregnancies, even allowing for the larger mothers. With the rising prevalence of type 2 diabetes and its emergence at younger ages, this is likely to become an increasingly important issue in coming years.

## 12.10 Which women should be screened for gestational diabetes, and how?

Screening and the exact criteria for diagnosis of gestational diabetes remain extremely controversial, with the USA and Australia generally espousing universal screening and lower 'normal' limits than the UK, Europe and New Zealand.

Current recommendations for the UK, Europe and New Zealand include:

■ urine testing for glycosuria at every antenatal visit
■ a random BG to be measured if glycosuria is detected

■ a 75 g oral glucose tolerance test (OGTT) if random BG is
>5.5 mmol/l fasting or >7.0 mmol/l 2 hours after eating
■ a routine 75 g OGTT to be performed at 28 weeks'
gestation.
Some regions with high proportions of patients from non-
European backgrounds are performing additional checks on high-risk
patients much earlier in pregnancy.

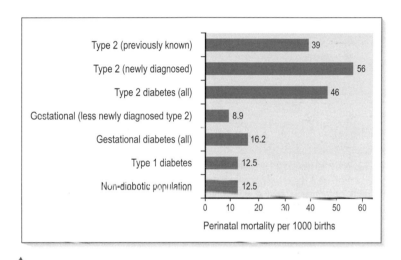

▲

**Fig. 12.1** Perinatal mortality in different groups with and without diabetes at National
Women's Hospital, Auckland (1985–1997).

## 12.11 Why do women with diabetes have large babies?

Many people will have heard that women with diabetes have large babies,
4.5 kg (10 lbs) or more – 'macrosomia'. This generally happens when the
glycaemic control during pregnancy is not ideal, though only totally normal
BG control would prevent it completely and this is not achievable with
current insulin treatment. Glucose crosses the placental barrier and
provides the foetus with nourishment. Maternal insulin does not cross the
placental barrier; however, from about 12 weeks of pregnancy, the foetal
pancreas becomes a functional endocrine organ. In the developing foetus,
the hormone insulin, as well as lowering PG, acts as a growth factor,
promoting fat deposition. Consequently, when the mother has diabetes, the
foetal pancreas responds to the raised PG and the resulting foetal

hyperinsulinaemia leads to fat deposition and macrosomia, particularly hepatomegaly.

### 12.12 What are the congenital abnormalities seen with diabetic mothers?

Most of the common renal, cardiac, neurological and skeletal abnormalities are increased two- to six-fold in most series, though caudal regression (e.g. sacral agenesis) is about 250 times more common, though still very rare. The most common abnormalities in practice are:

- cardiac
- skeletal (e.g. spina bifida or hemivertebra)
- neurological (e.g. microcephaly, anencephaly)
- renal (e.g. renal agenesis, duplex ureter).

The relationship with glycaemic control at the time of conception is clear – in one recent study those with HbA1c < 7.5% at booking had a major abnormality rate below 1% while those with higher values had a rate over 8%.[1]

### 12.13 Why does my patient with diabetes need to be seen so frequently during pregnancy?

Because of the multiple issues outlined above, women with diabetes in pregnancy need close supervision by the specialist obstetric and diabetic teams. Most units have developed a special joint clinic for these patients to ensure close liaison and see women with diabetes every 2 weeks for the duration of the pregnancy. For some women with problems, weekly visits are required with additional telephone contacts between visits. The aims of care are to:

- achieve excellent glycaemic control, with a normal HbA1c
- avoid severe hypoglycaemic episodes
- monitor foetal growth rate by ultrasound scans at 2-week intervals from 28 weeks' gestation
- detect any obstetric complications at an early stage
- plan delivery
- provide care and support for the woman with diabetes.

### 12.14 Is insulin always needed in gestational diabetes? Can't oral agents be used?

Insulin is not always needed but the issue here is obtaining *optimal* glycaemic control. If this can be done by diet and lifestyle measures, then no further treatment is needed. Unfortunately targets are often not achieved and insulin is frequently needed.

There has always been anxiety about the use of OHAs in pregnancy because some drugs such as gliclazide cross the placenta and lead to neonatal hypoglycaemia after delivery. Glibenclamide does not cross the placenta and was recently reported to be as safe as insulin in a randomised controlled trial in gestational diabetes in the US.[6] However, this has not gained wide acceptance in most centres.

The situation for metformin is less clear. This drug is being increasingly used before and during pregnancy in polycystic ovarian syndrome where it helps to induce ovulation and reduce miscarriage rate. The safety profile in this situation seems to be reasonable. A major study of metformin in gestational diabetes is underway, but at present OHAs are not recommended except by experienced specialists.

## 12.15 In which women should pregnancy be avoided?

The woman with diabetes needs an enormous commitment and high level of responsibility when considering pregnancy. It is critical that all women of reproductive age are made aware of this, so a personal informed choice can be made. Patients who struggle with diabetic management or suffer with hypoglycaemic problems, particularly lack of hypoglycaemic awareness, may be advised that pregnancy will place too large a burden on their daily living. Nevertheless, many women and their partners do proceed with a pregnancy, even though the risks are high and they are aware of them. Particular issues include retinopathy and nephropathy.

- ■ *Retinopathy*: Pregnancy is best avoided while patients have active sight-threatening retinopathy since pregnancy can aggravate retinopathy. However, with appropriate laser photocoagulation, many women can be successfully treated. Once the ophthalmologist feels a stable state has been achieved, pregnancy may be considered.
- ■ *Nephropathy*: Nephropathy as evidenced by persistent proteinuria carries high risks for mother and baby. Renal function may rapidly deteriorate in pregnancy and, if renal impairment is already present at conception, superimposed pre-eclampsia is common, necessitating early delivery and the risks of prematurity in the baby. There is also the mother's future health and probable reduced life expectancy, though this is not worsened by pregnancy.

## 12.16 Should women with diabetes be advised to have their children before they get too old?

Complications of pregnancy do tend to be commoner in older mothers, and some authorities recommend completion of the family by age 35, though this may not be the most important issue: duration of diabetes and presence of complications may be more relevant. If a young women with diabetes asks this question, you might discuss the likelihood of future complications based on her age at diagnosis, usual glycaemic control and presence of complications to date.

With a recently diagnosed patient you might advise her to consider having her pregnancies relatively soon if she has plans for a family. Residual pancreatic beta-cell function in the first 1–2 years of diabetes can often mean good glycaemic control and relatively easy management of diabetes in pregnancy. Ultimately it is for the patient to decide, based on the best information available to her.

## BREAST FEEDING

### 12.17 What about breast-feeding while on anti-diabetic medication?

Insulin use is safe, but both sulphonylureas and metformin are found in milk (albeit in small concentrations) and, as such, are contraindicated. This does sometimes cause real difficulties in patients with type 2 diabetes after pregnancy and some experts will permit low doses of metformin.

## HORMONE REPLACEMENT THERAPY

### 12.18 Is hormone replacement therapy safe for women with diabetes?

There had been a widely held belief in the medical profession that HRT was good for women because of the beneficial effects on lipids and the assumed reduction in cardiovascular disease. However, recent studies – WHI and HERS among others – have shown that HRT has significant detrimental effects in terms of increased risk of breast cancer and cardiovascular disease, only partially balanced by the benefits of increased bone density and reduction in colon cancer. Women with diabetes have a higher baseline cardiovascular risk than the general female population so HRT is likely to increase the risk further. Women with established coronary artery disease had an increased number of vascular events in the first year of HRT treatment compared with placebo.[7,8] In the light of the recent evidence, women with diabetes should not normally be recommended HRT when they reach the menopause.[9]

However, if a women with diabetes has significant menopausal symptoms or is at high risk of osteoporosis, HRT might be used for a short period after due consideration of the risks and benefits. Care needs to be taken in assessing the woman, as vascular disease in diabetes is often occult. Factors likely to increase risk of vascular events include hypertension, proteinuria, hyperlipidaemia, cigarette smoking or a family history of ischaemic heart disease or cerebrovascular accident. This needs to be carefully discussed with the patient.

HRT may lead to a slight deterioration in glycaemic control due to oestrogen affecting insulin action; a small increase in insulin or OHA dosage may be required. In some patients, blood pressure rises and lipids, particularly triglycerides, may deteriorate. Close monitoring should highlight any problems.

## SEXUAL FUNCTION AND IMPOTENCE

### 12.19 Does diabetes affect female sexual function?

This is a contentious issue, as indeed in the non-diabetic woman – some authorities consider this to be a 'non-disease' generated by the pharmaceutical industry. There is, however, some evidence and a possible mechanism for some rare instances of autonomic neuropathy causing a reduction in sexual pleasure and/or lubrication.

### 12.20 How common is impotence/erectile dysfunction among men with diabetes?

There is no doubt that men with diabetes, both type 1 and type 2, have a higher rate of erectile dysfunction compared with age-matched non-diabetic subjects, though the frequency of this varies widely with the definition and survey method – often self-reported.[10] Autonomic neuropathy is a major contributor, though vascular disease affecting the penis is often significant, especially in the older patient.

For type 2 diabetes, the excess risk is less – perhaps 30% – but the problem is still common. It appears that smoking, poor glycaemic control and other microvascular complications are all associated with the problem.

### 12.21 What are the usual causes of impotence?

The major contributors to erectile dysfunction are often multiple and include:

- Neurological causes: autonomic neuropathy
- Vascular causes: arterial disease
- Drugs: multiple antihypertensives – thiazides, beta-blockers
- Recreationals: excessive alcohol use, drug misuse (e.g. cannabis)
- Psychological causes.

Generally, longer diabetes duration, older age and the presence of other complications (nephropathy, retinopathy, peripheral neuropathy or macrovascular disease) make it more likely that organic disease is primarily responsible.

People with diabetes can, of course, have unrelated causes for erectile dysfunction such as hypopituitarism or hypogonadism, but these are rare unless there is a linking causative factor such as haemochromatosis.

## 12.22 How do I detect psychological causes of erectile dysfunction?

This remains largely a matter of clinical diagnosis, and is not specific to diabetes. Classically, the onset may be more abrupt and often related to home or work stress, depression or to relationship problems – libido is often affected as well. Intermittent symptoms, perhaps with a particular partner, and the preservation of early morning erections suggest non-organic causes.

While uncommon, a full history and examination is worthwhile to look for the issues described above, together with signs of general ill-health, endocrine and gonadal disease and cardiovascular status. This is important as individuals with psychological causes of impotence are much more likely to recover erectile function than those due to organic disease.

## 12.23 What investigations are necessary for erectile dysfunction?

Clinical examination will only occasionally give clues, for example signs of liver disease from alcohol/haemochromatosis, small testes, lack of body hair. In many cases where the features are typical of diabetes, no further investigations are needed, though the yield for hypogonadism is probably sufficient to justify this – it additionally demonstrates to patients that other causes have been sought. Where any of the differential diagnoses listed in *Question 12.21* need to be considered, then specific tests (e.g. liver function tests, thyroid function, testosterone, luteinising hormone/follicle stimulating hormone, prolactin) may be indicated and sometimes are needed to reassure patients that all possible avenues have been explored.

Where no cause is found and there is no indication of psychological causes, spontaneous improvement is uncommon.

## 12.24 What treatments are available for impotence?

There is now a range of treatments available for erectile dysfunction though none is universally successful. Most successful are the cyclic guanosine monophosphate phosphodiesterase inhibitors that extend the vasodilatory effect of nitric oxide. Sildenafil and similar agents increase the rate of successful intercourse by three- to five-fold (from 10–20% to 60–70%), the effects lasting for a few hours; the recently introduced tadalafil is claimed to last for 36 hours. They are *contraindicated* in patients taking nitrates and their use is complicated by vasodilatory problems such as headache, dizziness, flushing and, occasionally, syncope. Dose titration is needed.[11,12]

Other methods (*Table 12.3*) need expert training; penile prostheses are not recommended.

**TABLE 12.3  Treatments for erectile dysfunction**

| Treatment method | Agent |
| --- | --- |
| Oral agents | Sildenafil (Viagra) |
| | Tadalafil (Cialis) |
| | Vardenafil (Levitra) |
| | Apomorphine (Uprima) |
| Intra-urethral gel | Alprostadil (prostaglandin E1) |
| Intra-cavernosal injection | Alprostadil |
| | Papaverine |
| | Phentolamine |
| Physical means | Vacuum devices |
| Surgery | Penile prostheses |

The choice requires extensive discussion with the patient and, ideally, their partner. Many patients will try a therapy but may not persist with its use, or use it only occasionally. While for many this is an issue of cost, for others it is not.

 **PATIENT QUESTION**

### 12.25  What is the likelihood of diabetes developing in my children?

Many pregnant women worry that the baby will be born with diabetes – this virtually never occurs.

- *Type 1 diabetes*: If the mother has type 1 diabetes, the chance of a child developing diabetes is low: approximately 3 in 200 offspring will develop diabetes by the age of 25 years. Even if both parents have type 1 diabetes, the risk is still only that around 1 in 20 children (5%) develop it. Only 10% of people with type 1 diabetes have a first-degree relative with the condition. In these families, the chance of a child developing diabetes is somewhat higher. One study has shown that the risk of offspring developing diabetes is greater if the father has type 1 diabetes rather than the mother (6% versus 1–2%). These risks are all surprisingly low – many prospective parents expect an answer of 1 in 4 or 1 in 2 (25% or 50%).

- *Type 2 diabetes*: In this situation, inheritance is generally a stronger influence and the chance of children *eventually* developing type 2 diabetes is higher. But it is still unusual for the onset of diabetes to be in childhood or adolescence, though this is sadly becoming commoner in non-European patients, especially where both parents already have diabetes. Avoiding the development of obesity will reduce the risk.

# Macrovascular disease and its prevention

# 13

## CARDIOVASCULAR DISEASE

### 13.1 Surely microvascular complications are more important than macrovascular disease?

No. Most deaths in people with diabetes are due to heart disease, though only in the past 10–20 years has this become clear from several long-term cohort studies.[1-4] The role of the diabetes and primary care physician has changed from a 'blood sugar' focus, predominantly on type 1 diabetes, to that of 'preventative cardiologist' for everyone with diabetes. This is not to reduce the importance of good glycaemic control in prevention of diabetes complications, micro- and macrovascular. The best outcomes in the UKPDS were in the group with *both* good glycaemic *and* good BP control.

### 13.2 What about macrovascular disease in type 1 diabetes?

This occurs later in the course of type 1 diabetes than many of the microvascular problems, unless nephropathy is present when it is often extremely premature – coronary artery disease (CAD), cerebrovascular and peripheral arterial disease at age 30–50 years (*see Ch. 1*). This is presumably because clinical arterial disease becomes apparent later in these young individuals, who may already have had 15–25 years of hyperglycaemic exposure in their thirties, but at least started with healthy vessels.

In contrast, those with type 2 diabetes, while presenting with diabetes later, may well have had atheroma in their young adult years caused by 'metabolic syndrome', impaired fasting glucose (IFG) and/or impaired glucose tolerance (IGT) and possibly undiagnosed diabetes.

### 13.3 How much commoner is heart disease in diabetes than in the general population, and why?

Many studies confirm substantial increases in the incidence and prevalence of CAD in people with both type 2 and type 1 diabetes.[2] The mortality mainly occurs after many years of diabetes (*Fig. 13.1*).

Most studies show a two- to five-fold increase in CAD, myocardial infarction (MI), sudden death, heart failure, stroke, peripheral arterial disease and amputation. Generally, CAD appears clinically more severe in people with diabetes and has a higher mortality. For example, mortality following MI and stroke is about double that of a matched non-diabetic population, and mortality following coronary surgical procedures is also significantly higher.

Only part of the excess is explained by known risk factors such as hypertension, dyslipidaemia and obesity. Other possible factors potentially contributing include:

- presence of the 'metabolic syndrome'
- diabetic nephropathy, including microalbuminuria
- possible 'diabetic cardiomyopathy', with diastolic dysfunction
- haemostatic factors, plasminogen activator inhibitor 1, fibrinogen and other clotting factors
- other biochemical risk factors (e.g. homocysteine, C-reactive protein)
- vascular calcification.

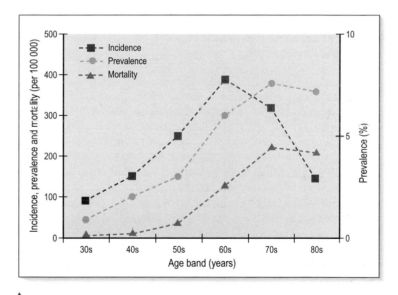

**Fig. 13.1** The time relationship between incidence, prevalence and attributable mortality in diabetes (data from New Zealand[5]).

### 13.4 Are people with diabetes aware of their increased risk?

No, not adequately – multiple studies report that most people with diabetes have little appreciation of their high risk for heart attack and stroke; indeed often they have no concept at all.[6] Education about this is essential to motivate appropriate participation in their own care and to explain the multiple medications they are prescribed. While fear should play no part in this (and does not appear to work anyway), proper information about the risks involved and their optimal treatment is a basic patient right (*see Q.13.56*).

### 13.5 Are any groups at particularly high risk?

Yes. First, women with diabetes have a very much higher risk of CAD than the general population. In the past this was commoner in type 1 diabetes than in European type 2, but is now changing as the latter is diagnosed earlier and is very relevant in many Asian, Afro-Caribbean, Maori and Pacific Island patients.

Second, renal disease, even microalbuminuria, considerably increases the risk of cardiovascular disease. While substantial, this is not as marked as in type 1 diabetes where patients with proteinuria have 50–100 times increased mortality compared to the general population (*see Ch. 14*).

Young people with type 2 diabetes as part of the 'metabolic syndrome' are of particular concern (*see Q. 1.12*). Apart from diabetes they may also have hypertension, dyslipidaemia, microalbuminuria and other features placing them at high vascular risk from their teens or twenties onwards.

### 13.6 Is the increased risk true for stroke as well as coronary artery disease?

Yes. Many studies show a two- to four-fold increased rate of stroke in people with type 2 diabetes.[7–9] This has previously been underestimated, as stroke tends to occur at older ages than CAD. With better data and longer survival of people with diabetes, stroke has become a more significant cause of mortality and morbidity. The excess is due to an increased incidence of thrombotic and ischaemic stroke, but not haemorrhagic events (*see Fig. 13.2*).

Additionally most studies show an increased mortality rate among people with diabetes following a stroke. Concern among patients about stroke, especially a disabling one, is often greater than about a heart attack.

### 13.7 How is life expectancy affected in patients with diabetes?

Survival figures still show substantial reductions in life expectancy for both type 1 and type 2 diabetes despite recent improvements in treatment. The

---

**BOX 13.1  Example of 'absolute' and 'relative' risks in a 4-year randomised controlled trial**

1. Control/placebo group: 1000 patients (400 strokes or heart attacks)
2. Wonder drug group: 1000 patients (200 strokes or heart attacks)

- The *absolute risk* of an event is therefore 10% per annum (400/1000 × 4) in the control group and the *relative risk reduction* for the wonder drug group is 50% (200/400).

- The *absolute risk reduction* is 400 − 200 over 4 years = 50 per 1000 patients per year = 0.05 (5%).

- The *number needed to treat* is the number of patients that need to be treated to prevent 1 event which is 20 (few interventions achieve this).

---

major cause of premature death is CAD, though stroke is increasingly important in older age groups.[1,10]

The reduction in life expectancy is greatest for those with type 1 diabetes, type 2 diabetes diagnosed at younger ages and again for those with nephropathy. Exact estimates are, by definition, out of date for current patients, and cardiovascular event rates in several current studies are substantially below the predicted figures, suggesting significant improvements in outcomes already, compared with those of even 10 years ago.

---

### 13.8  What exactly do the 'absolute' and 'relative' risks in papers refer to?

These are best illustrated by the example in *Box 13.1* of an imaginary randomised 4-year trial of a 'wonder drug' in patients with diabetes.

### THE UNDERLYING PATHOLOGY

### 13.9  Are there any pathological differences in the arterial disease seen in diabetic and non-diabetic patients?

While some studies demonstrate no convincing differences, others show that individuals with diabetes have more diffuse CAD, involving frequently both proximal and distal arteries with multiple rather than single diseased arteries and segments. Surgeons frequently complain at the small calibre of arteries they are required to suture in patients with diabetes.

The same data are not so clear for cerebrovascular disease, though there is increasing evidence of carotid arterial endothelial thickening in diabetes and, indeed, in metabolic syndrome. Recent studies have shown that this may be prevented by good control.

### 13.10 Are there any new theories of the pathogenesis of arterial disease?

Yes. Most important is the discovery of significant inflammatory components in the pathogenesis of atherosclerosis (though this is not specific to diabetes), thus the finding that the inflammatory marker C-reactive protein (CRP) may be useful in risk assessment (*see Q. 13.54*).[10,11]

Also, many ischaemic events are clearly caused by unstable plaque in coronary arteries rather than by total physical occlusion of the lumen.[12] The action of aspirin may be helpful in this area. It is postulated that some of the actions and benefits of statins, fibrates and glitazones may be on these processes, rather than just on circulating levels of plasma lipids.

### 13.11 Are there differences in the presentation or outcome of arterial disease in type 2 diabetes?

This is hard to study because of potential selection bias: those with type 2 diabetes are often under regular medical supervision. There are strong suggestions that more have silent ischaemia, painless MI and atypical symptoms of ischaemic heart disease than those without diabetes. It is prudent to treat chest pain, breathlessness or other possible symptoms of CAD with a high level of suspicion in type 2 diabetes, especially in those from non-European backgrounds. Unusual symptoms with a lack of chest pain should also alert the physician.

Worryingly, patients with type 2 diabetes appear to present later when unwell with acute episodes of CAD, possibly related to the frequent atypical range of symptoms. Physicians often see people with diabetes admitted just generally unwell and, 24 hours later, see ECG or enzyme evidence of MI. This may mean that thrombolytic treatment is not given.

## RISK FACTORS FOR CARDIOVASCULAR DISEASE IN DIABETES

### 13.12 What are the major risk factors for coronary and cerebrovascular disease in diabetes? Do these differ from people without diabetes?

Much evidence demonstrates that the major coronary risk factors – hypertension, smoking and dyslipidaemia – are also valid in diabetes.[13,14] Poor glycaemic control is also associated with more cardiovascular disease as seen with MI in the UKPDS[15] (*see Fig. 2.4*). In middle-aged and elderly patients with diabetes and hypertension, there is evidence that intervention may be particularly effective in reducing relative and absolute risk.

### 13.13 What is the best risk factor calculation method to use?

The Framingham equation has been used for many years, but its significant limitations must be recognised. It was derived from a cohort of individuals in a US town 40 years ago, of whom only 337 had diabetes, predominantly but not exclusively type 2.[16,17] The particular problems are:

- it is a US historical cohort, nearly all of European ancestry
- the small total number with diabetes, with no account of type or duration
- glycaemic control could not then be measured
- recent studies suggest that it may underestimate risk in diabetes, and overestimate elsewhere.

Recently a modern calculation has been derived from UKPDS data, including both duration of diabetes and glycaemic control (*Box 13.2*).[18] It too has limitations, being strictly applicable only to a geographically limited UK population with newly diagnosed type 2 diabetes. It does, however, separate the coronary and stroke risks, and can calculate these over any given time period, but requires validation in other populations.

### 13.14 Are there any limitations to these risk factor methods?

Unfortunately lots  – *see Q. 13.13* and additionally:

- They apply to risks calculated from *untreated levels* of BP and lipids.
- They may not apply to other ethnic groups, though the UKPDS included Afro-Caribbean and Asian groups. Younger and elderly patients were not included.

---

> **BOX 13.2  Risk factor calculation for cardiovascular disease in diabetes**
>
> - The UKPDS Risk Engine is a program developed specifically for calculating the risk of coronary heart disease in individuals with type 2 diabetes. It incorporates diabetes-specific variables and gives an approximate 'margin of error' for each estimate.
> - It provides risk estimates for both coronary heart disease and stroke in individuals with type 2 diabetes not known to have heart disease. These can be calculated for any given duration based on current age, sex, ethnicity, smoking status, presence or absence of atrial fibrillation and levels of HbA1c, systolic blood pressure, total cholesterol and high density lipoprotein cholesterol.
>
> *See www.dtu.ox.ac.uk.*

■ They normally apply to individuals who have *not* already developed cardiovascular disease.

■ They are invalid for individuals with other specific high-risk pathologies:
— familial dyslipidaemias
— diabetic nephropathy (or indeed renal dysfunction of any cause).

■ They underestimate risk for:
— long-standing and/or poorly controlled diabetes (Framingham)
— recent smokers – risk will lie between current and non-smoking values
— those with metabolic syndrome, IGT or IFG
— those with strong family histories of premature coronary heart disease (CHD)
— people with type 1 diabetes
— women with premature menopause.

### 13.15 Should we use 5- or 10-year risks? Coronary or total cardiovascular risk?

Different authorities use different time intervals and event outcomes. All have strengths and weaknesses, which are not important as long as like is being compared with like.

Calculations over long periods are an average, exaggerating risk in the early years while underestimating it in later ones, particularly important for 10-year calculations. A broad comparison of the outcomes used is given in *Table 13.1*.

Obviously the Framingham model gives higher risks; in general, a 15% 5-year Framingham risk approximates to a 20% 10-year coronary risk, but the relative importance of stroke and heart failure increases with age (*see Fig. 13.2*). The British Joint Societies coronary risk prediction is still derived from the original Framingham cohort data and is not based on UK subjects.

| **TABLE 13.1  Comparison of coronary and cardiovascular risk in diabetes** | |
| --- | --- |
| **British Joint Societies** *Coronary risk prediction* | **Framingham-based models** *Cardiovascular risk equation* |
| New angina | New angina |
| Non-fatal myocardial infarction | Non-fatal myocardial infarction |
| Coronary death | Cardiovascular-related death |
| | Ischaemic stroke |
| | Transient ischaemic attack |
| | Congestive cardiac failure |
| | Peripheral vascular disease (claudication) |

## 13.16 How about the risks in the elderly?

As people get older, risk is dominated by age rather than by BP or lipids; predicted risk will always be high, however 'healthy' these readings. An example is given in *Figure 13.2* for UKPDS and Framingham calculations: here any diabetic patient over 70–75 years is classified as 'high risk'.

With increasing age, a tension develops between the absolute risk-based epidemiological view, suggesting ever-increasing treatment, and the working clinician approach.

## 13.17 What about younger patients with apparent single risk factors?

Younger patients with apparent single risk factors (e.g. hypertension or hypercholesterolaemia) is an area that leads to profound disagreement between epidemiologists and public health physicians who deal with *populations*, and clinicians who deal with real *individuals*. Many of these individuals do not reach levels of *absolute risk* where treatment would be

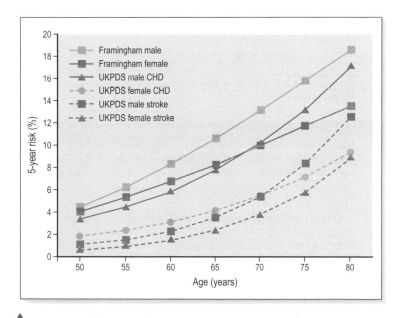

**Fig. 13.2** Comparison of risk method calculations: Framingham male and female values and the separate UKPDS coronary and cerebrovascular (stroke) risk values with increasing age for a hypothetical patient in whom the only change is age. Note the powerful effect of age and the increasing importance of stroke. CHD, coronary heart disease.

recommended, while clinicians would consider they should be for potential personal benefit, for example:

- A 42-year-old Asian man with type 2 diabetes for 5 years has a total cholesterol of 7.2 and high density lipoprotein (HDL) of 1.0 mmol/l but good glycaemic control, good BP and no other risk factors. His UKPDS CHD 10-year risk is only 11–12%, but most physicians would treat him with a statin.
- A 50-year-old lady, with a 5-year history of diabetes, has BP of 165/100 mmHg but healthy lipids and no other risk factors. Her calculated 10-year risk is around 5%, yet most clinicians would not countenance leaving her hypertension untreated.

To be fair to the guidelines, most specifically say that they do not apply to these situations and that calculators should not over-ride clinical judgement.

### 13.18 Can these equations be used for patients already receiving treatment?

Strictly, no. Untreated initial levels for BP and lipids should be used, and smoking is a yes/no answer. That said, there is no alternative method, but any such calculated value is only a very rough guide. Changes in the actual levels of risk factors achieved on treatment are probably more valuable, especially for BP – but obviously this does not work for aspirin use or for smoking cessation!

### 13.19 Is it true that having type 2 diabetes is as big a cardiovascular risk as already having had a myocardial infarction?

This is controversial. It arose from a 1998 Finnish study of a cohort of patients in the 1980s to 1990s,[10] but has not been confirmed in more recent studies based on community-recruited populations nor in the recent Heart Protection Study (*Fig. 13.3*).[19,20]

Two current large-scale lipid-lowering trials (CARDS and FIELD) are reporting cardiovascular event rates well below those initially predicted, which in turn are below those reported in the Finnish study. These may have excluded higher-risk patients, so the truth probably lies in between. As a personal view, it may be best to regard people with type 2 diabetes as potentially 'high risk' unless they can be shown to be otherwise.

### 13.20 How sensitive are the usual detection methods for coronary and cerebrovascular disease?

Unfortunately, risk factor calculations are more useful for population measures than for individuals. As in the non-diabetic population, the majority of infarcts occur in those with relatively 'normal' levels of BP or

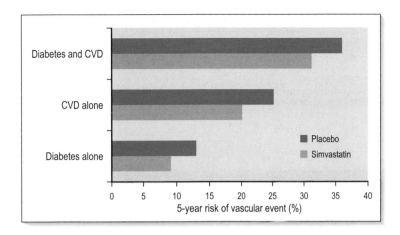

**Fig. 13.3** Event rates in the Heart Protection Study: the event rate in the diabetes group without known cardiovascular disease (CVD) is substantially less than the non-diabetic group with known heart disease. Those with diabetes and CVD have the highest rate. (Adapted from Heart Protection Collaborative Study Group[20] with permission from Elsevier.)

cholesterol. To alter population outcomes significantly, it is necessary to reduce the overall risk factors of the population rather than targeting only those who have high absolute risks.

Specific issues for diabetes include the following:

■ Early clinical symptoms are often absent, so many individuals present with a first fatal MI or stroke. Those presenting with new angina, unstable angina and transient ischaemic attacks should be treated rapidly and energetically as they have a worse and premature outcome.
■ A normal resting ECG does not exclude significant CAD.
■ Exercise testing with ECG monitoring can be a useful way of detecting asymptomatic CAD.
■ Echocardiograms can be helpful in identifying left ventricular hypertrophy and heart failure, both common in diabetes.

## 13.21 How important is smoking in vascular risk in diabetes?

Most epidemiological studies show the usual expected relationship between smoking and cardiovascular disease.[21,22] There are obviously no randomised trials of smoking cessation!

Unfortunately, significant numbers of patients with type 2 diabetes continue to smoke. Techniques for aiding cessation of smoking can be used in diabetes, though amfebutamone (Zyban) is only recommended at a lower dose because of the risk of precipitating convulsions with hypoglycaemia. Provided the patient does not have significant coronary, cerebral or peripheral arterial disease, nicotine products such as Nicorette can be useful in coping with the smoking addiction problems. In the UK and many other countries, specific services to help smoking cessation have been established and diabetic patients who smoke would benefit from referral (*see also Appendix 2*).

## LOWERING CARDIOVASCULAR RISK

### 13.22 How do I assess the need for intervention? Do I treat individual 'diseases/risk factors' or the overall level of risk?

This requires a total individual assessment, but most national advisory bodies now recommend a risk calculation (*see Qs 13.13–13.15*) as the primary guide to the level of intervention (*see Case vignettes 13.1–13.3*).

### 13.23 Are there any exceptions?

Yes. As discussed above (*see Qs 13.16–13.18*) several groups of patients are at high risk simply on clinical grounds and should be energetically treated without the need for a calculation. These include:

■ individuals with known macrovascular disease of any type
■ those with a familial dyslipidaemia
■ patients with nephropathy including microalbuminuria or, to a lesser extent, renal dysfunction from other causes (*see Ch. 14*).

Calculated levels also underestimate risk for several other groups (*see Q. 13.14*).

The increased cardiovascular risk for people with type 1 diabetes is recognised. Treatment with aspirin and a statin is advised from 35 years of age unless the patient is at high risk due to renal disease or there is a strong family history, when earlier intervention is recommended.

### 13.24 Are pharmaceutical treatments always needed?

Not always, but usually is the honest answer. Lower levels of risk are managed with lifestyle modification, though this should already be the case for people with type 2 diabetes. Dietary salt reduction may have an additional small benefit in those who are hypertensive (*see Q. 13.29*).

## 13.25 Which interventions are easiest, most beneficial and cost-effective?

> This is controversial – some would say all patients above a given threshold should receive optimised glycaemic control, smoking cessation advice if needed, energetic anti-hypertensive therapy, low-dose aspirin and lipid-lowering therapy.
>
> ■ *Good glycaemic control* is hard to achieve in many patients but has widespread beneficial effects on all adverse outcomes in diabetes. The reduction in macrovascular outcomes in UKPDS was disappointing as was the HbA1c reduction of 0.9%, but that translates to a reduction of approximately 14% in the MI event rate for each 1% reduction in HbA1c. For *macrovascular risk alone*, it is an expensive economic option based on life-years saved.[23]
>
> ■ *Smoking cessation* is cheap, effective but difficult to achieve – it has beneficial effects in reducing the risk of other diseases such as lung cancer as well as cardiovascular outcomes.[24]
>
> ■ *Anti-hypertensive* treatment is simple to start and cost-effective. Indeed, in several studies it is cost-saving when drug costs are balanced against the reduced number of cardiovascular events.[23] However, in people with diabetes three to four drugs are often required to achieve either target BP or at least optimal levels.[25]
>
> ■ *Aspirin* is cheap, easy to start and take, and is extremely cost-effective.[26,27]
>
> ■ *Lipid-lowering* therapy is simple but relatively expensive (i.e. drug costs).[20,23]
>
> If economic concerns are predominant, smoking cessation, anti-hypertensive treatment and aspirin currently have the best cost:benefit ratio for this purpose.

## 13.26 How energetic should I be in tackling risk? How much can it be reduced?

Most guidelines recommend pharmacological treatment for patients above a given risk level, aiming to reduce as far as possible. Generally the higher the absolute risk, the greater the benefit from treatment.

One recent study in high-risk patients with microalbuminuria showed a 50% risk reduction with intensive treatment (3-monthly specialist follow-up, strict glycaemic control, aggressive anti-hypertensive treatment, lipid-lowering therapy and aspirin),[28] and theoretical models suggest up to 75–80% of the risk may be reduced.[29]

## 13.27 Do all the interventions act independently?

This is an important question, difficult to answer completely as most major trials are done with simple interventions. It does appear that the main interventions are independently beneficial so that multiple treatments will produce incremental (though not multiplicative) improvements in outcome (*see Case vignettes 13.1–13.3*).

---

### 13.28 What do people with diabetes see as worthwhile risk reductions if it means taking even more tablets?

Surprisingly little research has been done in this area. A recent landmark study indicated that British patients have higher expectations of drugs than their doctors.[30] Most wanted an absolute risk reduction of $\geq$ 20% in order to take it for 5 years, and to be told the numerical benefit expected. Most interventions fall way short of this efficacy.

---

## INCREASED BLOOD PRESSURE

### 13.29 How should 'hypertension' or raised blood pressure be treated?

Simple lifestyle advice should already have been given but may need repetition; the same measures recommended for control of diabetes will improve BP and lipid profile (e.g. weight loss if needed, a healthy diet, avoiding excess salt, increased physical exercise; *see also Ch. 4*). There are numerous clinical trials on the importance of intensive hypertension treatment in type 2 diabetes,[31] such as UKPDS, HOT, SHEP, SystEur, ALLHAT, ABCD (*see Glossary*).

Basically, treatment of hypertension with any agent that achieves systolic BP reductions of >10 mmHg will reduce cardiovascular events and microvascular complications (*Table 13.2*). Choice of agents is discussed in *Questions 13.32–13.36; see also Case vignettes 13.1–13.3*.

---

### 13.30 What should the threshold or target pressures be? Or should there be a specific target?

The BP level at which drug treatment should commence is unclear, and indeed absolute risk rather than BP level is now used as the main guide. Benefit is undoubted at $\geq$160/100 mmHg but, at 140/80 to 159/89 mmHg, there is less clear evidence unless nephropathy is present. Specifically, the National Institute for Clinical Excellence (NICE) guidelines recommend that all those with BP persistently $\geq$160/100 mmHg should receive treatment. The recent British Hypertension Society guidelines for hypertension management 2004 (BHS-IV)[32] suggested a threshold of 140/90 mmHg and a target of <130/80 mmHg for everyone with diabetes (*Table 13.3*), thus continuing a trend towards even lower targets.

**TABLE 13.2  A guide to choice of drug class for blood pressure control in diabetes**

| Accompanying problem | Major advantages | Choice of agent | |
|---|---|---|---|
| | | Advantages | Contraindications, Disadvantages, Precautions |
| **Diabetes** | | | |
| Diabetes alone | | Low-dose thiazides ACE inhibitors A2 receptor blockers Beta-blockers Calcium antagonists | High-dose thiazides |
| Proteinuria Microalbuminuria | ACE inhibitors Some calcium antagonists A2 receptor blockers | | |
| Renal impairment | | | Potassium-sparing agents |
| **Cardiovascular disease** | | | |
| Angina | | Beta-blockers Calcium antagonists | |
| Myocardial infarction | Beta-blockers ACE inhibitors | | |
| Heart failure | ACE inhibitors Diuretics Beta-blockers | | Verapamil/diltiazem (CI) |
| Peripheral arterial disease | | Beta-blockers Some calcium antagonists | Beta-blockers (CI) |
| Atrial fibrillation | | | |
| **Other conditions** | | | |
| Asthma/COPD | | | Beta-blockers (CI) |
| Depression | | | Beta-blockers |
| Gout | | | Diuretics |

CI, contraindicated; COPD, chronic obstructive pulmonary disease.

## 13.31 Is the systolic, diastolic or pulse blood pressure more important?

Previously the main emphasis in diagnosing and treating hypertension related to diastolic BP. Systolic BP is now recognised as more important. Epidemiological studies show the strongest relationship between

**TABLE 13.3 Overview of recent guideline blood pressure targets (where given)**

| Guideline | Target systolic BP (mmHg) | Target diastolic BP (mmHg) | With renal disease (mmHg) |
|---|---|---|---|
| SIGN 2001 | <140 | <80 | <140/80 |
| NICE type 2 diabetes mellitus | <140 | <80 | <135/75 |
| ADA 2003 | <130 | <80 | <130/80 |
| NZGG 2003: | As low as possible towards 115/70 mmHg but specifically: | | |
| Those with cardiovascular disease | <130 | <80 | <120/75 |
| Those at lower risk | <140 | <85 | <120/75 |
| BHS 2004 | Start if ≥ 140/900 mmHg | | <130/80 |
| | <130 | <89 | |

cardiovascular events, mortality and *systolic* pressure. In the UKPDS, the incidence of MI increased by 11% for each 10 mmHg increment in systolic BP above 120 mmHg (*see Fig. 2.4B*).

Isolated systolic hypertension, previously thought unimportant, needs treatment in all age groups. There is indeed good evidence that wide pulse pressure (systolic BP–diastolic BP) is a bad prognostic sign, indicating inelastic arteries. So, at a given systolic BP, those with *lower* diastolic BP carry *higher* risk.

## 13.32 Which agents should be used and in what order?

The choice of agent depends upon many factors, and there is no simple algorithm. Since the results of ALLHAT, most authorities would regard thiazide diuretics and angiotensin converting enzyme (ACE) inhibitors as the preferred first-choice agents when possible, i.e. a 'Premier Division', with calcium antagonists and beta-blockers close behind in the 'First Division' (*Box 13.3*).

There is some evidence that alpha-blockers may not be as beneficial as other agents, and generally little long-term evidence for the Step 3 drugs.

The particular benefits and problems of groups of drugs in different groups of patients are listed in *Table 13.2*.

> **BOX 13.3 'Steps' in the administration of anti-hypertensive agents in diabetes**
>
> ■ Step 1:
> — ACE inhibitors (A2RA if not tolerated)
> — thiazide diuretics (low-dose)
> ■ Step 2:
> — beta-blockers
> — calcium antagonists, non-dihydropyrridine (verapamil and diltiazem)
> — calcium antagonists, long-acting dihydropyrridine
> ■ Step 3:
> — furosemide (frusemide) instead of thiazide, especially if renal impairment
> — addition of A2RA to ACE inhibitor
> — centrally acting agents
> — alpha-blockers

## 13.33 What are the particular pros and cons of angiotensin converting enzyme inhibitors in diabetes?

Multiple trials have shown major benefits of ACE inhibitors in subgroups of patients with renal disease, microalbuminuria or high vascular risk (*Table 13.2*). The ALLHAT study showed no superiority, and some inferiority.[33 36] They may have marginal positive effects on glucose tolerance, with several reports in hypertension trials of significant protection against the subsequent development of diabetes in ACE inhibitor-treated groups.

Side effects appear similar to those in non-diabetic patients, commonest being a dry cough in around 10%, often overlooked. Others are rashes, loss of taste and, rarely, angio-oedema. They can cause hyperkalaemia and impairment of renal function; serum creatinine and electrolytes should be checked before and 5–10 days after starting. A small increase in serum creatinine ($\leq 25$–40 $\mu$mol/l) is common and not a cause for concern. They should not be used where renal artery stenosis is suspected – concern about renal function warrants specialist referral.

## 13.34 What are the pros and cons of beta-blockers?

Beta-blockers were long avoided in diabetes because of concern that they mask symptoms of, and impair recovery from, hypoglycaemia. In practice this is rarely a problem. The UKPDS showed that they matched an ACE inhibitor for beneficial effect but were less well tolerated. They have a particular role in patients with CAD and have their many usual limitations.

The hypoglycaemia issue is really only a problem with type 1 patients with frequent hypoglycaemia and/or unawareness. Much greater limitations are patients with asthma and the other side effects: only selective beta-blockers should be used.

## 13.35 What about calcium antagonists? Aren't there problems in diabetes?

Some initial studies certainly indicated that the dihydropyrridine calcium antagonists (e.g. amlodipine, felodipine) were less effective in preventing heart failure but this has since been largely dispelled by larger studies. Nifedipine should not normally be used. Verapamil and diltiazem are effective agents, though evidence on diltiazem as an anti-hypertensive is weak. Both need to be used with caution (if at all) with conduction disorders or heart failure, but may have advantages in patients with renal disease.

There is a widespread feeling (but little evidence) that dihydropyrridines demonstrate more side effects, particularly oedema, in patients with diabetes than in the non-diabetic.

## 13.36 What are the pros and cons of diuretics?

The findings of ALLHAT, that low-dose thiazides were as effective and well tolerated as newer agents, came as a surprise to many. The study has been criticised, but certainly shows that, for many, they are a cheap and effective agent, especially in the elderly and those of African extraction where some other agents work less well. Physiologically, hypertension in diabetes is associated with sodium retention, so perhaps the results are not such a surprise.

Some specific side effects such as gout and impotence are important. But thiazide diuretics now form the backbone of many regimens – in particular with the ACE inhibitor where the combination once-daily tablets undoubtedly have advantages in adherence.

Their place in the metabolic syndrome is less convincing as they cause or aggravate uric acid levels, lipid profiles, hypokalaemia and the development of diabetes. ALLHAT may not have been long enough to detect all their long-term problems.

Loop diuretics, largely furosemide (frusemide), are used when renal function is impaired and a greater natriuresis is required – in general they are only effective as anti-hypertensive agents in the presence of an ACE inhibitor or angiotensin 2 receptor antagonist (A2RA).

## 13.37 How about angiotensin 2 receptor antagonists?

If these had come first, ACE inhibitors wouldn't have stood a chance! In general, there is little difference as far as hypertension treatment is concerned but angiotensin 2 (A2) blockers are expensive, though extremely well tolerated. They are most often prescribed in situations where ACE inhibitors are not tolerated, especially due to the cough.

Combination therapy with both ACE inhibitors and A2 blockers appears extremely promising in non-diabetic renal disease,[37] though in diabetic nephropathy this should currently be confined to specialists (*see Q. 14.11*).

### 13.38 How about other anti-hypertensive agents?

These are summarised in *Table 13.2*. There is little, if any, evidence on which to make a choice, which is usually determined by patient characteristics, tolerability and effectiveness when used.

## ANTI-PLATELET THERAPY

### 13.39 Should every diabetic patient be on low-dose aspirin?

There are wide differences between countries and clinicians in this area. Overall, low-dose aspirin reduces the cardiovascular event rate by 15–30% (relative risk), with a small attributable increase in haemorrhagic stroke and gastrointestinal bleeding. The consensus is that those with a 10-year coronary risk above 15% will benefit from aspirin, assuming no contraindications.[26,27] However, American recommendations are more aggressive, current guidelines suggesting that all diabetic patients over 30 should be treated.

A reasonable primary prevention approach Is for aspirin therapy if 10-year coronary risk is ≥ 15%. Patients with existing cardiovascular, peripheral arterial or cerebrovascular disease or at high risk because of hypertension and/or renal disease should be treated with aspirin unless contraindicated (*see Case vignettes 13.1–13.3*).

Aspirin is extremely cheap and very cost-effective.

### 13.40 What is the correct dose of aspirin in diabetes?

Trials show no real difference between doses of 75 and 300/325 mg/day. There are theoretical reasons from platelet studies, though no hard data, why people with diabetes may need higher doses than others, so some clinicians use 100–300 mg/day rather than 75 mg.

### 13.41 What are the risks of aspirin therapy? Are there alternatives?

These are no different to the non-diabetic population. They relate to rare intracerebral bleeding and a marginally increased risk of haemorrhagic stroke found in some, but not all, studies and the usual gastric bleeding which can occur even at low doses. Absolute benefit increases with the absolute cardiovascular risk. There is widespread agreement that hypertension should be controlled before aspirin treatment is commenced – NICE guidelines recommend reducing systolic BP to 145 mmHg or less.

Clopidogrel or ticlopidine are alternative agents though there are fewer data available in people with diabetes. They may be used where aspirin is contraindicated or not tolerated but have more limitations and side effects than aspirin, are expensive and should at present only be started by specialists.

## LIPID-LOWERING THERAPY

### 13.42 What is the evidence for use of lipid-lowering therapy in diabetes?

The dyslipidaemia in type 2 diabetes is not generally just about high total or low density lipoprotein (LDL) cholesterol levels. Often, especially with the metabolic syndrome, these levels are not particularly high but involve a more complex series of typical changes:

■ low HDL levels
■ raised triglycerides
■ 'normal' LDL cholesterol
■ raised total cholesterol:HDL ratio
■ more small dense LDL particles which are particularly atherogenic.

The evidence for therapy in patients with *established* coronary artery disease and diabetes is overwhelming from subgroup analyses of many studies, and now most importantly from the Heart Protection Study in which vascular events were reduced by about 25%.[14,38–41]

Statin studies include the 4S study, CARE, WOSCOPS, LIPID and HPS; for fibrates, HHS, HIT and DAIS[42] (*see Glossary*).

These studies demonstrate that statin therapy produces a benefit of about 20–30% in reduced mortality and cardiovascular event rates. There are few long-term outcome studies for fibrate therapy, except for the HIT study that showed 20–25% benefit for gemfibrizol in patients with low HDL.[43] However, fibrates may be particularly effective in patients with the metabolic syndrome and diabetic dyslipidaemia as they increase HDL levels and lower triglyceride levels.

### 13.43 Is the evidence as good for 'primary' prevention of cardiovascular disease?

The evidence was not so persuasive or consistent but has recently been strengthened. The Heart Protection Study[20] recently published their results of 6000 patients with diabetes (*Fig. 13.4*). Patients were aged 40–80 years with total cholesterol >3.5 mmol/l. They were randomised to simvastatin 40 mg daily or placebo and followed for 5 years; there was a 25% reduction in first event rate, even if there was no pre-existing CAD and irrespective of the initial cholesterol level; lipid changes were as outlined in *Table 13.4*.

Additionally the CARDS atorvastatin study, about to be published, has demonstrated roughly a 35% reduction in cardiovascular events.

The main consideration for primary prevention may relate to the level of absolute risk and the cost of lipid-lowering intervention.[23] At present it is reasonable to undertake a risk calculation in all diabetic patients aged >35–40 years to determine whether to treat, with active treatment in those

### TABLE 13.4 Heart Protection Study: lipid changes

|  | Change | Reduction/increase (%) |  |
|---|---|---|---|
| Total cholesterol | 5.7 to 4.6 | reduction of 1.1 | (– 18%) |
| LDL cholesterol | 3.2 to 2.3 | reduction of 0.9 | (– 28%) |
| HDL cholesterol | 1.06 to 1.07 | increase of 0.01 | (+ 1%) |
| Triglyceride | 2.3 to 2.0 | reduction of 0.3 | (– 13%) |

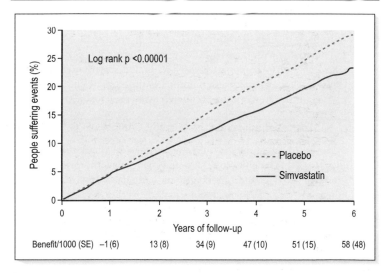

**Fig. 13.4** Results of Heart Protection Study diabetes group: first major vascular event according to treatment allocation to simvastatin or placebo. SE, standard error. (From Heart Protection Collaborative Study Group[20] with permission from Elsevier.)

at high risk, say >15% risk over 10 years; this threshold may fall (*see Case vignettes 13.1–13.3*).

When future studies report, particularly the FIELD cohort which examines fibrate treatment, the situation should become clearer.

## 13.44 What are the advantages and disadvantages of statins?

Statins work by inhibiting a hepatic enzyme involved in cholesterol synthesis (HMG CoA-reductase). They are potent in reducing total and LDL cholesterol levels with a small reduction in triglyceride levels (*see Q. 13.42*).

Clinical evidence is best for simvastatin, pravastatin and atorvastatin. Rosuvastatin is a promising new agent with impressive biochemical changes but, as yet, no hard outcome data. Approximate LDL reductions on 40 mg daily of each agent are:

- atorvastatin: 45–55%
- fluvastatin: 25–30%
- lovastatin: 35–40%
- pravastatin: 25–30%
- rosuvastatin: 50–55%
- simvastatin: 35–40%

 In general statins show similar tolerability to the non-diabetic population. Side effects include gastrointestinal upset, disordered liver function tests and myopathy with raised creatine kinase. Some patients complain of vague aches and pains when treated with a statin: it is important to check creatine kinase levels, as these are often normal so the patient can be reassured and advised to continue treatment. Rhabdomyolysis is fortunately rare.

## 13.45 How about the fibrates?

Evidence for the fibrates is much weaker than for the statins but growing (*see Q. 13.42*). The HIT study showed benefit of gemfibrozil in patients with low HDL levels, greatest in the diabetic and metabolic syndrome subgroups.[43] The DAIS angiographic study has also shown reduced coronary narrowing after treatment with fenofibrate[42] while the FIELD study, largely of primary prevention in low-risk patients, will complete in 2005.

There is increasing interest in the combination of low-dose statins and fibrates, which appear to be synergistic in their effect on lipid patterns and to be well tolerated.

 Side effects of fibrates include gastrointestinal upsets and renal function changes, together with a myopathy usually indicated by painful muscles and accompanied by a rise in creatine kinase.

### 13.46 What other lipid-lowering agents can I use?

There are multiple other agents including fish oils, resins, acipimox and nicotinic acids. They are difficult to use and poorly tolerated, especially in diabetes – they should be left to specialists!

Ezetimibe is a promising new cholesterol-absorption agent, potentially useful when statins are not tolerated or not fully effective. The combination of a low dose statin plus ezetimibe is as effective in lowering cholesterol as a high dose statin. As yet there are no outcome data.

## OTHER INTERVENTIONS

### 13.47 Is smoking cessation valuable?

Yes. Most reports of smoking cessation programmes show only a small proportion of patients giving up smoking permanently. However, the benefit to these people is substantial and all patients should be actively encouraged to stop.[22] Doctors and health professionals need to promote cessation; when smoking is not actively discussed, patients may perceive that the doctor thinks that it is acceptable in their case. This is obviously far from the truth! (*See also Q. 13.21 and Appendix 2.*)

### 13.48 Should people with diabetes receive an ACE inhibitor anyway?

The HOPE study considered high-risk cardiovascular patients, including 3600 with diabetes.[44] Ramipril (10 mg daily) or placebo was added to existing medication, resulting in 20–25% risk reductions in cardiovascular death and MI but minimal change in BP in both diabetic and non-diabetic groups. There were additional benefits in prevention of nephropathy. Therefore it is recommended that all high-risk patients should receive an ACE inhibitor as part of their treatment, though it is surprising that the ALLHAT study did not show similar benefit. A very low dose ACE inhibitor may not be effective and therefore a full dose ACEI is essential to gain benefit.[45]

The LIFE study with an A2RA found a similar advantage.[46] This trial compared losartan with atenolol in the treatment of hypertension: losartan was superior despite similar falls in BP, though by a lesser margin than in the HOPE study which was placebo controlled.

### 13.49 Are there are any differences in cardiovascular prevention treatment for people with type 1 diabetes?

Cardiovascular disease is the major cause of death in type 1 diabetes after the early years where ketoacidosis, hypoglycaemia and accidents

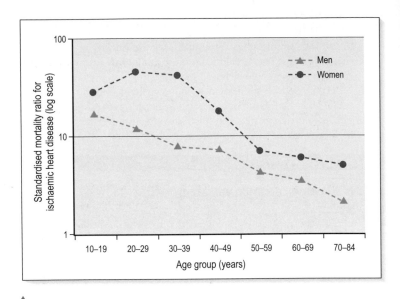

**Fig. 13.5** Standardised mortality rates for ischaemic heart disease in men and women with insulin-treated diabetes (mainly type 1 diabetes) diagnosed below age 30 (drawn from data in Laing et al.[1]). Note the massively high relative rates, especially for pre-menopausal women.

predominate (*Fig. 13.5*).[1] Relative risk is massively increased, but absolute risk is still low unless the patient has nephropathy.

There are relatively few data applicable to those with type 1 diabetes without nephropathy, and little recent cohort data on life expectancy and cardiovascular mortality.

It is reasonable (but unproven) to commence an ACE inhibitor, aspirin and, possibly, lipid-lowering treatment when the patient reaches around 40 years of age, sooner if there is a strong family history of CAD (*see Q. 13.23*).

New guidelines from NICE on the management of type 1 diabetes will be published during 2004.

## 13.50 Is it possible to summarise the evidence and strategy?

Hard, but *Table 13.5* shows one interpretation of the evidence for the different interventions on macro- and microvascular risk.

The strategy now is to use multiple risk-reducing therapies, aiming to reduce overall risk rather than just individual factors.[47]

**TABLE 13.5  Interventions on macro- and microvascular risk**

*Macrovascular disease*

| Intervention | Coronary risk | Stroke risk |
|---|---|---|
| Improved glycaemic control | + | + |
| Blood pressure reduction | +++ | +++ |
| Lipid lowering | +++ | +/++ |
| Aspirin | ++ | + |
| ACE inhibition | + | + |

*Microvascular disease*

| Intervention | Retinopathy | | Nephropathy | | Neuropathy |
|---|---|---|---|---|---|
| | Prev. | Progr. | Prev. | Progr. | |
| Improved glycaemic control | +++ | +++ | +++ | +++ | ++ |
| Blood pressure reduction | ++ | ++ | ++ | ++ | ? |
| Lipid lowering | ? | ? | ? | ? | ? |
| Aspirin | 0 | 0 | ? | ? | ? |
| ACE inhibition | ? | ? | ++ | +++ | ? |

Prev., Prevention; Prog., Progression; +++, strong beneficial effect; ++, clear beneficial effect; +, some beneficial effect; 0, no or minimal effect; ?, insufficient or inadequate data.

## ESTABLISHED CARDIOVASCULAR DISEASE

### 13.51 Does management of coronary artery disease differ in diabetes from other patients?

Essentially no, except for a higher threshold of suspicion and lower threshold for intervention/referral. Unfortunately, patients with diabetes seem to take longer to get hospital treatment after suffering a MI, and receive less in the way of intervention than they should. Particular points are:

- Thrombolytic therapy should be given with the usual indications. The theoretical risk of a retinal haemorrhage from diabetic retinopathy is totally insignificant beside the mortality benefit.
- Beta-blockers are not contraindicated in diabetes (*see Q. 13.34*).
- Too few patients are given low-dose aspirin after a MI.
- Given the double mortality post-MI, specialist follow-up is recommended.

### 13.52 Is there any evidence that intensive insulin therapy is beneficial in myocardial infarction or similar situations?

Mortality from MI in diabetes is double that of non-diabetic patients, despite equal-sized infarcts, but there have been conflicting data from intervention trials.

The Swedish randomised DIGAMI study has shown an 11% *absolute* mortality reduction from immediate and continuing insulin treatment in patients suffering a MI, though there are some inconsistencies in the data.[48] Many clinicians now recommend intensive insulin infusion treatment for all type 2 and type 1 diabetic patients in the acute situation.

Use of intensive insulin treatment *after* recovery from the MI remains controversial. Many specialists adopt a pragmatic approach, using twice-daily pre-mixed insulin therapy where glycaemic control was previously inadequate.

The situation with acute stroke is uncertain. Again mortality rate in diabetes is doubled in stroke, and controlled trials of insulin infusions during the acute phase are underway. Higher BG levels after acute stroke are associated with increased mortality, and some stroke units are using intensive regimens while trial results are awaited.

### 13.53 Is surgical treatment of coronary artery disease different in diabetes?

In general, cardiac intervention in diabetes (whether angioplasty, bypass surgery or heart transplant) is somewhat less successful than in the non-diabetic patient, but differences are relatively small and reducing with time. People with diabetes are often not referred for surgery because of this perception which may, in turn, be creating the problem. For primary care and indeed for the specialist physician, diabetes should make no difference to the decision to refer.

Glycoprotein IIb/IIIa inhibitors such as abciximab are used in specialised cardiac situations.

## NEWER RISK FACTORS

### 13.54 What about newer factors such as hs-CRP and homocysteine in diabetes?

Many new risk factors have been proposed in recent years; the most important are summarised in *Table 13.6*. At present, there is no evidence that measuring or monitoring levels of these risk factors is useful in everyday practice, though high-sensitivity C-reactive protein (hs-CRP)

**TABLE 13.6  Newer risk factors in diabetes**

| Test | Comments |
|------|----------|
| High-sensitivity C-reactive protein[11] | Excellent correlation with cardiovascular risk, better than LDL cholesterol<br>No evidence yet on treatment effect |
| Homocysteine[49] | Some evidence of relation with cardiovascular risk<br>Treatment with folate lowers homocysteine; no firm evidence yet of benefit with folate supplements |
| Lipoprotein (a), apolipoproteins | Some predictive value, but difficult to modify |
| Small dense LDL | Fairly specific to diabetes/metabolic syndrome<br>No evidence yet of modification leading to benefit |
| Oxidants | Good theoretical case but clinical trials of antioxidants (e.g. vitamin E etc.) have proved entirely negative |

appears to be as good a predictor of cardiovascular outcome as LDL cholesterol.

## FUTURE DEVELOPMENTS

### 13.55 What future developments are likely in cardiovascular protection in diabetes?

The following are probable:

- More precise risk assessments as arterial biology is better understood. Non-invasive tools may allow earlier delineation of vascular disease, and hence targeting of individual treatment.
- New agents will include novel anti-hypertensive drugs, also lipid-lowering agents that can halt or potentially reverse progression of atheroma.
- Combination pills including several different classes of agents have been developed; one UK team recently suggested that all adults over 55 should take one of these with three anti-hypertensive agents: a 'statin', aspirin and folic acid – the 'polypill'.[29]

### CASE VIGNETTE 13.1

A 51-year-old man with type 2 diabetes is well controlled on metformin 850 mg twice daily, HbA1c 6.8%. He presents with recent intermittent claudication, and Doppler scan confirms a significant stenosis in the right superficial femoral artery warranting referral to a vascular surgeon. His BP was 156/88 and 150/92 mmHg at the last two checks. Should this be treated?

*Comment*

He is likely to have coronary artery as well as peripheral arterial disease. Useful investigations would include ECG, echocardiogram and exercise testing. With evidence of macrovascular disease (claudication), this is secondary prevention and he is at >20% 10-year risk. His BP is high and should be treated. If there is renal disease, even microalbuminuria, or if left ventricular hypertrophy is evident, an ACE inhibitor would be the first-line drug, though serum creatinine *must* be checked after 5–10 days to check for atherosclerotic renal artery stenosis. Otherwise, a thiazide diuretic would be an equally good choice but not a beta-blocker (claudication). The treatment aim would ideally be a systolic BP ≤130 mmHg. He also requires anti-platelet therapy with aspirin and a statin, irrespective of current cholesterol level.

### CASE VIGNETTE 13.2

A 74-year-old woman with type 2 diabetes for 5 years has hypertension on ramipril 10 mg daily. She has no history of macrovascular disease and no evidence of nephropathy. Glycaemic control is good on metformin 500 mg twice daily, HbA1c 6.1%. Total cholesterol (TC) is 5.6 mmol/l, LDL cholesterol 3.6 mmol/l, TC:HDL ratio 5.1. Recent BPs have been 154/86, 168/92 and 160/76 mmHg. Is this treatment adequate and/or what else should she be receiving?

*Comment*

Her current 10-year risk is over 30% and her anti-hypertensive treatment is not achieving 140/80 mmHg, a reasonable target even in older patients. Reduction should be gradual, but the long-term goal remains the same as the absolute risk is higher in the elderly, and so is benefit of treatment.

Next is probably a low-dose thiazide diuretic, for example, bendroflumethiazide (bendrofluazide) 1.25–2.5 mg daily. After this, choices would be a beta-blocker and/or a calcium antagonist assuming no contraindications. Whilst many patients do need four different agents to control BP, it would be surprising here as levels are not excessively high. Check adherence and the understanding of need for treatment.

Otherwise, BP measurements at home or undertaking a 24-hour BP monitor might be useful. Once BP is under control, aspirin should be added. She should probably also be on a statin.

### CASE VIGNETTE 13.3

A 56-year-old man with type 2 diabetes is on simvastatin 10 mg daily following a recent MI. His glycaemic control is good on diet alone, HbA1c 5.9%. BP is 116/74 mmHg. His fasting lipid profile shows total cholesterol (TC) 5.4 mmol/l, triglyceride 3.1 mmol/l, LDL cholesterol 4.1 mmol/l, HDL cholesterol 0.8 mmol/l and TC:HDL ratio 6.8. What more should be done?

*Comment*

This man is on a statin but his lipid profile has not reached the post-MI target levels of TC <5 mmol/l or LDL of ≤2.6 mmol/l. The dose of simvastatin is modest and should probably be increased to 40 mg (as in HPS[20]). As he has high triglycerides and low HDL levels which respond relatively poorly to statin treatment, further benefit might be gained by adding a fibrate (e.g. fenofibrate). He will need to have the treatment monitored and be warned about the possibility of myopathy – though this is less now that cerivastatin has been withdrawn.

He should also presumably be receiving (unless contraindicated) aspirin, a beta-blocker and an ACE inhibitor.

---

 **PATIENT QUESTION**

### 13.56 Does diabetes really increase my risk of heart disease, and what can be done about it?

Yes, it does, but the risk can be substantially reduced. This often hasn't been well enough explained by doctors in the past but all studies clearly show that heart attacks and strokes have been commoner in people with diabetes, and occur earlier.

Several recent large studies have shown that better blood pressure control and the use of aspirin, special blood pressure drugs (the ACE inhibitors) and cholesterol (lipid)-lowering drugs all reduce this risk, and there is increasingly good evidence that people with diabetes are living much longer than previously.

It is also true that the physically fit and healthy-eating groups live longer.

Discuss this with your own team; it's helpful if you understand how you can personally cut down your risks and what all the 'targets' and drugs are.

# Renal disease in diabetes

## FUTURE CHANGES

### PQ PATIENT QUESTIONS

## DEFINITIONS, PATHOLOGY AND DIAGNOSIS

### 14.1 What are the definitions of diabetic renal disease, microalbuminuria and overt diabetic nephropathy?

Diabetic renal disease is a clinical condition of altered renal function accompanied by structural changes in the kidney. It progresses through a continuum of hyperfiltration and renal hypertrophy, increased protein excretion to declining renal function leading to end-stage renal failure. Diabetic renal disease and its subsequent progression are associated with several risk factors, of which hyperglycaemia, raised BP, smoking and dyslipidaemia are open to intervention. It is frequently associated with other diabetic microvascular complications, and carries a substantially increased risk of macrovascular disease.

- *Microalbuminuria*: This is defined as *persistent* urinary albumin excretion between 30 and 300 mg/day. A good estimate is provided by the urinary albumin:creatinine ratio (ACR), with values ≥2.5 mg/mmol in men and ≥3.5 mg/mmol in women indicating microalbuminuria. An equivalent threshold on a timed urine collection is approximately 20 mcg/min.
- *Clinical/overt diabetic nephropathy*: This is defined by *persistent* urinary albumin excretion ≥300 mg/24 hours, corresponding to clinical proteinuria as reliably detected by albumin dipstick (e.g. Albustix). An equivalent ACR on a random urine sample is about 25 mg/mmol.

### 14.2 What actually happens to the kidney?

This is summarised in *Table 14.1*: it is important to realise that this is a continuum.[1,2] The pathology is of initial basement membrane thickening in

| TABLE 14.1 The progressive changes with diabetic nephropathy | |
|---|---|
| **Progressive changes (1–6)** | **Status** |
| 1. Normal | GFR normal (e.g. 100 ml/min) |
| | BP normal (e.g. 120/80 mmHg) |
| | Well |
| | Albuminuria <20 mg/day |
| 2. Hyperfiltration | Increased GFR (e.g. 120 ml/min) |
| 3. Microalbuminuria | Albumin excretion 30–300 mg/day |
| | Marginal increase in BP (e.g. 130/80 mmHg) |
| 4. Persistent proteinuria | Progressive increase in proteinuria, albumin >300 mg/day |
| | Progressive increase in BP (e.g. 140/90 mmHg) |
| | Progressive linear reduction in GFR |
| | Initial rise in serum creatinine, often within normal range |

the glomerulus that leads to altered pressures and function within the glomerular capillaries causing leakage of proteins, particularly albumin. In the early stages many of the abnormalities are reversible but, eventually, increasing glomerular damage leads to scarring, permanent loss of function and dramatically increasing proteinuria. As renal damage occurs, hormonal changes in the kidney lead to raised BP, which appears to amplify the damage process and the amount of proteinuria.

The stage of microalbuminuria (also known as 'incipient nephropathy') is not normally associated with any reduction in renal function, as measured by glomerular filtration rate (GFR) or serum creatinine, but serves as a warning that the pathological process has begun (*Fig. 14.1*).

### 14.3 How is diabetic nephropathy diagnosed?

The pathological diagnosis can only be confirmed on a renal biopsy, but the clinical features and investigations are usually so typical that this is rarely needed. The characteristic histological lesions are diabetic glomerulosclerosis (the Kimmelstiel–Wilson lesion of old textbooks) and mesangial thickening. The hallmark features of established nephropathy are outlined in *Box 14.1*.

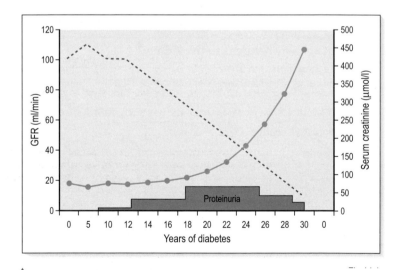

**Fig. 14.1** The natural history of diabetic nephropathy, showing changes in proteinuria, glomerular filtration rate (GFR) and serum creatinine. Note that significant renal function (GFR) is lost while the serum creatinine remains little changed within the normal range.

---

**BOX 14.1 Hallmark features of established nephropathy**

■ At least 5–10 years of diabetes (including before diagnosis in type 2)
■ Continuous significant proteinuria
■ Mild–moderate increase in blood pressure
■ Rarely any other finding in the urine; haematuria, cells and casts are uncommon
■ Normal- or large-sized kidneys on ultrasound
■ Usually significant retinopathy, but not always in type 2 diabetes, especially if non-European

---

Other causes of renal disease can be present in people with diabetes, and sometimes both exist together (e.g. diabetic nephropathy and long-term previous essential hypertension). Basic investigations such as urine culture and renal ultrasound need to be undertaken to exclude other treatable causes including:

■ renal disease long preceding diabetes
■ essential hypertension
■ renal stone disease
■ gout

■ congenital abnormalities
■ glomerulonephritis
■ pyelonephritis.

Patients with single kidneys (congenital or surgically removed) appear to be more vulnerable to nephropathy.

## RISK AND SCREENING

### 14.4 What are the main risk factors for diabetic nephropathy?

These are, in rough order of importance:
■ *Glycaemic control*: Those with long-term poor control show higher rates of nephropathy and all other microvascular complications.[3]
■ *Ethnicity*: Non-European populations consistently appear to have a higher rate of nephropathy.
■ *Family history/genetics*: This is important, and occasionally seen dramatically in family pedigrees, though the underlying genetic factor is not well defined. Raised blood pressure may be part of the mechanism.
■ *Adherence*: Almost all studies demonstrate that non-compliant/non-adherent individuals have outcomes similar or worse than the poorest-controlled but compliant patients.
■ *Smoking*: Most but not all studies show higher rates of nephropathy, and more rapid progression, in smokers.

■ *Specialist input*: This is one of the few areas where evidence suggests that specialist follow-up produces better patient outcomes than generalists or primary care.
■ *Male gender*: Nephropathy appears to occur more commonly in men than in women, especially in type 1 diabetes.

### 14.5 Is diabetic nephropathy commoner in any particular ethnic groups?

There is strong evidence that many non-European groups have very high rates of end-stage diabetic nephropathy including specifically South Asian, African–American, Afro-Caribbean, Maori, Pacific Island and Australian aboriginal groups. This does not appear to be explained entirely by later diagnosis or less good care of diabetes, though this may often play a role.[4] It also tends to occur at a younger age.

### 14.6 What is the chance of developing microalbuminuria or diabetic nephropathy? Is it changing?

Early studies suggested 30% of individuals with type 2 diabetes go on to develop some degree of diabetic nephropathy, though many older patients will die of unrelated or related causes long before it develops. Even with nephropathy, major cause of death in type 2 diabetes is cardiovascular disease as shown in *Figure 14.2*.[5]

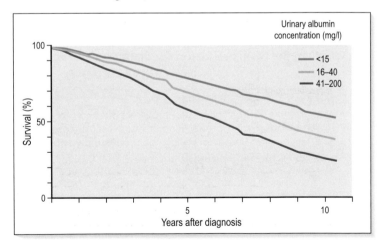

**Fig. 14.2** Microalbuminuria as a risk factor for death in type 2 diabetes. (From Schmitz and Vaeth[5] with permission from Blackwell Publishing.)

For some people, microalbuminuria or proteinuria will be present at diagnosis as many years of undiagnosed hyperglycaemia have elapsed. Microalbuminuria is unlikely before 5 years of actual (not diagnosed) type 2 diabetes and the highest chance appears to be between 10 and 25 years' duration; it rarely develops in patients who survive over 30 years with no problem.

Studies from Scandinavia and the USA in type 1 diabetes show the incidence of nephropathy is falling over successive cohorts of patients diagnosed in the 1960s to 1980s.[6] Whether the renal damage has been prevented or simply delayed is not yet known. The likely reason for the reduction is improved care of diabetes with tighter glycaemic and BP control. While it does not follow that this is also true in type 2 diabetes, most studies show very similar patterns between the two types.

In the UKPDS the following transitions were observed in newly-diagnosed patients in the 10 years after diagnosis:[7]

■ No nephropathy:
   ↓           *2.0% per annum, 25% after 10 years*
■ Microalbuminuria:
   ↓           *2.8% per annum, 5% of all after 10 years*
■ Macroalbuminuria:
   ↓           *2.3% per annum, 0.8% at 10 years*
■ Serum creatinine:   *>175 μmol/l or renal replacement treatment*

Progressively higher cardiovascular mortality was seen in the affected cohorts (*Fig. 14.3*).

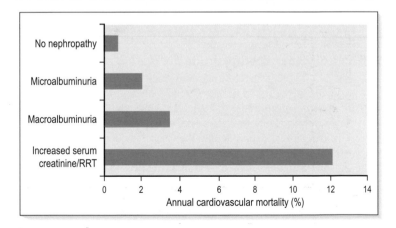

▲

**Fig. 14.3** Increasing cardiovascular mortality at progressive stages of diabetic renal involvement in type 2 diabetes. RRT, renal replacement therapy. (Data from UKPDS[7] with permission from Blackwell Publishing.)

### 14.7 Who should be screened for diabetic renal disease, how often and with what method?

A simple dipstick test for proteinuria (e.g. Albustix) may be positive, implying significant proteinuria and the need for full investigation. If this is negative or unavailable, measurements of urinary albumin provide the most sensitive screening test. There is considerable day-to-day variability in urinary albumin excretion so an abnormal result requires a repeat test for confirmation.

Patients with type 2 diabetes should be screened at diagnosis with annual checks thereafter. A first morning urine specimen is most reproducible, though not always practicable; a random sample for estimation of the ACR is also acceptable. The latter calculation corrects for variable dilution of the urine, and allows a reasonable estimation of daily urine albumin excretion.

Laboratory methods are preferred to near-patient tests, though the latter may be acceptable where laboratory tests are unobtainable or inconvenient. A single normal value in a first morning urine sample confirms normo-albuminuria, but the definition of microalbuminuria or overt nephropathy requires confirmation in two or more of three samples.

Serum creatinine should be measured annually. The reference range is wide, and renal function, as measured by GFR, may deteriorate substantially while serum creatinine increases within the 'normal' reference range (*see Fig. 14.1 and Table 14.1*). GFR can be estimated from serum creatinine as outlined in *Box 14.2*.

Non-proteinuric renal impairment is now recognised (*see Q. 14.17*).

### PREVENTION AND TREATMENT

### 14.8 Can diabetic nephropathy be prevented?

The DCCT, UKPDS and Kumamoto studies all showed a substantial reduction in the risk of developing microalbuminuria, proteinuria and rising serum creatinine with better glycaemic control (*see Q. 2.3*). Subsequent epidemiological analysis of the UKPDS cohort suggested that, with every 1% HbA1c reduction, the chance of developing nephropathy and retinopathy was cut by about 35%.

The UKPDS also showed that reducing BP (154/87 to 144/82 mmHg) was associated with a decreased risk for developing microalbuminuria. The epidemiological analysis suggested a risk reduction of about 12% for each 10 mmHg decrease in mean systolic BP, with no lower threshold (*see Fig. 2.4B*).

**BOX 14.2 Estimating glomerular filtration rate**

An approximate value for creatinine clearance and glomerular filtration rate (GFR) can be derived as follows from:

- serum creatinine in μmol/l
- weight in kg
- height in cm
- age in years.

Creatinine clearance (ml/min) for:

males    = 1.23 × weight × (140 − age)/creatinine
females  = 1.04 × weight × (140 − age)/creatinine

Thus, for a 50-year-old man of weight 70 kg with a stable serum creatinine of 115 μmol/l:

creatinine clearance    = 1.23 × 70 × 90 ÷ 115
                        = 67.4 ml/min (significantly reduced).

For an average-sized person this is an adequate method, but for very large or small individuals a correction is needed to give a truer picture of GFR:

$$\text{GFR (ml/min/1.73 m}^2) = \frac{\text{creatinine clearance} \times \text{body surface area}}{1.73}$$

Body surface area is derived from widely available nomograms, or there are on-line calculators for GFR at *www.nephron.com.*

## 14.9 What is the optimal treatment for patients with overt nephropathy?

Several recent studies have shown that intensive BP control reduces the rate of adverse outcomes, including death, vascular events such as myocardial infarction and need for renal support (dialysis or transplant) in patients with nephropathy. The target BP for optimal effect is 125/75 to 130/80 mmHg. There appears to be additional benefit from ACE inhibitors (ACEI) and angiotensin 2 (A2) blockers over other anti-hypertensive agents,[8–10] though no study has compared ACEI and angiotensin 2 receptor antagonist (A2RA) directly. Maximal therapeutic doses of these agents are needed and, generally, several anti-hypertensive agents are needed to approach target BP levels (*Fig. 14.4*). A recent trial (COOPERATE) in non-diabetic renal disease suggests that dual therapy with both ACEI and A2RA further reduces progression;[11] though not yet replicated in diabetes, studies measuring BP and proteinuria support this contention.

Smoking has been associated with an increased prevalence of diabetic nephropathy and more rapid progression once established.[12] All patients should be strongly encouraged to stop (*see Appendix 2*).

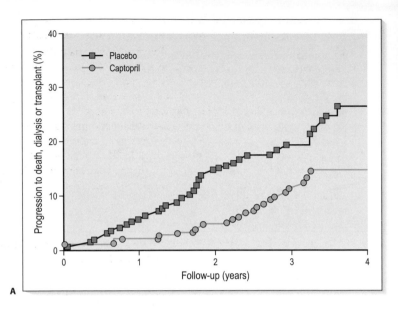

A

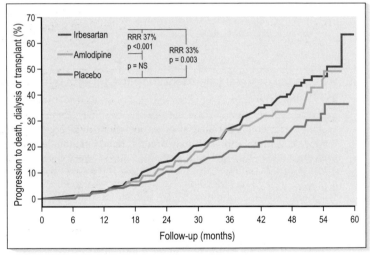

B

**Fig. 14.4 A**, Effect of angiotensin converting enzyme inhibition on progression of nephropathy in patients with type 1 diabetes, with benefit to captopril compared with placebo. *p = 0.006 versus placebo. **B**, Time to doubling of serum creatinine in the IDNT study with benefit to irbesartan compared with amlodipine or placebo. NS, not significant; RRR, relative risk reduction. (Adapted from Lewis et al.[8,9] Copyright © 1993, 2001 Massachusetts Medical Society.)

## 14.10 Should all patients who have microalbuminuria be treated?

Essentially yes, though obviously not all microalbuminuria is due to diabetes (*see Q. 14.3*). Treatment with an A2RA or ACEI reduces the rate of progression to overt nephropathy – *this is still the case even when BP is not obviously raised.*[13,14] While these studies depend on the use of the surrogate end-point of proteinuria, the latter appears to be a good marker of intrarenal progression of the disease process. Comparison dose studies suggest that the maximum dose of these agents (e.g. enalapril 20–40 mg/day, irbesartan 300 mg/day) be given for optimal protection, though they produce relatively little BP change in normotensive patients. Recent studies have shown that energetic multifactorial treatment can halve cardiovascular events[15] (*see also Q. 14.12*).

## 14.11 What are the risks associated with ACE inhibitor or A2 blocker treatment in patients with diabetic renal disease?

In those with overt diabetic nephropathy, institution of any BP lowering treatment often produces a decline in renal function, usually small, that probably relates to loss of autoregulation of renal blood flow. Serum creatinine and potassium should be checked about 5–7 days after starting patients on treatment or after a large dose increase (e.g. enalapril 5 to 40 mg/day)

A small rise in serum creatinine is predictable in the short term and, in general, a rise of 20–40 µmol/l is not an indication to withdraw therapy. The drop in renal function with ACE inhibitors or A2 blockers may be greater because of their intrarenal mechanism of action, but a diagnosis of renal artery stenosis should be considered if a marked creatinine rise is seen.

Hyperkalaemia is an occasional side effect of ACE inhibitor or A2 blocker treatment, aggravated by other potassium-retaining drugs (e.g. amiloride, spironolactone). It may occur as renal function deteriorates even with a relatively modest rise in serum creatinine – dietary potassium reduction or diuretic addition is sometimes necessary: serum potassium should be checked regularly in all patients on these agents.

## 14.12 What other treatment should patients with microalbuminuria or overt nephropathy receive?

Because of the high risk of macrovascular disease and premature mortality with worsening renal disease, these individuals require intensive management of other risk factors (*see Fig. 14.3*).[7,16,17] Treatment should include low-dose aspirin for its vascular protective action, and ACE inhibitor or A2RA therapy (if not already included in hypotensive medication), probably plus statin therapy for lipid lowering.[15] For those with impaired renal function, drugs such as non-steroidal anti-inflammatory agents should be avoided.

These patients are also at much increased risk of other microvascular complications and require frequent screening especially for macular oedema (type 2), proliferative retinopathy (especially type 1) and peripheral and autonomic neuropathy (*see Case vignette 14.1*).

Beyond microvascular complications, they have multiple unfavourable cardiovascular risk factors including dyslipidaemias, abnormal clotting factors and left ventricular hypertrophy and dysfunction which lead to very high rates of coronary artery, cerebrovascular and peripheral vascular disease.

Issues such as dietary protein restriction and renal bone disease are beyond the scope of this book.

## CASE VIGNETTE 14.1

This patient has been known to have type 2 diabetes for 11 years with indifferent control (HbA1c of 8–9.5%) until recently when he has become more interested in his care, since a relative died following an amputation. He is currently taking metformin 1 g b.d. and enalapril 5 mg daily. On annual review you note the trend in his results as outlined in *Table 14.2*.

*Comment*

Both his BP and ACR are increasing, suggesting progressive renal damage. Indeed his serum creatinine is also rising in the later years (though still within the 'normal' range). While he is correctly on an ACE inhibitor, the dose is inadequate – full doses are needed for maximal anti-hypertensive and renoprotective action. Enalapril 20–40 mg (or other ACE inhibitor) would be recommended with the addition of a low-dose thiazide or furosemide (frusemide) if needed to achieve a BP of 125/75 mmHg or below. Moreover, his glycaemic control should be improved and a full vascular risk assessment conducted – he will need low-dose aspirin and/or statin therapy.

Additionally he is more likely to have retinopathy and/or neuropathy than a patient without nephropathy, and will need more frequent follow-up and biochemical monitoring than annually.

### TABLE 14.2 Changing trends on annual review in type 2 diabetes

| Year | BP (mmHg) | Albumin:creatinine ratio (mg/mmol) | Serum creatinine (µmol/l) |
|------|-----------|-------------------------------------|----------------------------|
| 1999 | 134/78 | 4.1 | 76 |
| 2000 | 138/76 | 8.6 | 75 |
| 2001 | 146/82 | 13.5 | 78 |
| 2002 | 144/88 | 17.7 | 81 |
| 2003 | 146/92 | 31.0 | 87 |

## DIABETES AND RENAL SPECIALIST ADVICE

### 14.13 When should these patients be referred to a diabetes or renal specialist?

In the past, patients were frequently referred too late to initiate treatment to reduce renal disease progression. These patients have the highest risk of mortality/morbidity of any subgroup in diabetes.

All patients with overt nephropathy should be referred to a diabetologist to optimize treatment and set up a long-term management plan. There is mounting evidence that intensive treatment of hypertension and the other risk factors in this situation is best achieved by specialists, though a shared care plan is often the best option. Most diabetologists and renal physicians work in close co-operation in a joint clinic or with an agreed protocol between the two specialties. Consensus recommendations for referral to a renal specialist unit include the following:

- Serum creatinine ≥150 µmol/l or calculated GFR < 60 ml/min/m$^2$.
- When the exact diagnosis of renal disease is in doubt.
- When there are rapidly increasing levels of microalbuminuria or proteinuria.
- When there is difficulty in achieving BP targets.

For type 2 diabetes with confirmed microalbuminuria, a recent Danish study reported that 3-monthly specialist review, with an intensive multifactorial package (intensive glycaemic control, anti-hypertensives, statin therapy and aspirin), produced a 50% reduction in the vascular event rate, compared to similar patients having conventional care in the community.[15]

### 14.14 When do these patients need renal replacement therapy?

It is generally accepted that patients with diabetic nephropathy tend to become symptomatic and tolerate renal impairment less well than patients without diabetes as the underlying cause. Most nephrologists will initiate preparations for dialysis or transplant well before a patient becomes symptomatic. It is essential to provide education and support in advance of the need for surgical, vascular or peritoneal access procedures.

### 14.15 What method of renal replacement treatment is best?

Choice of renal replacement treatment (RRT) method varies between patient groups, countries and different centres. Patients with type 2 diabetes are more likely to have cardiac disease which often limits survival and affects choice of method. Many people also have other problems such as blindness or amputations, which limit both their suitability for RRT and the

TABLE 14.3  Renal replacement treatment: advantages and disadvantages

| Treatment | Advantages | Disadvantages |
|---|---|---|
| Transplant | One-off treatment | Limited supply of organs, lifetime immunosuppression |
| Continuous ambulatory peritoneal dialysis | Applicable to most, easier training | Access problems, infections, adequacy of dialysis |
| Haemodialysis | More effective than peritoneal dialysis | Expensive equipment/staff, inflexible timing, ? greater cardiac stress |

choice of method. The main advantages and disadvantages for each method are outlined in *Table 14.3*.

Full assessment by the renal team and discussion of the options with the patient, family and carers are essential for the best decisions to be made.

## 14.16 What is the prognosis for patients with diabetic nephropathy?

The major cause of death, both before and after RRT, is coronary artery disease, not renal failure itself.[7] Thus optimal care requires attention to multiple risk factors (*see Q. 14.12*), not just the progression of renal disease. The previously extremely high mortality and morbidity rates have been substantially reduced in recent clinical trial cohorts involving energetic anti-hypertensive treatment and multifactorial interventions.

Unfortunately patients with diabetes survive less well on RRT than patients without diabetes, though there have been encouraging trends in improved survival in recent years, particularly for patients with type 2 diabetes.

## 14.17 What is non-proteinuric renal failure and how common is it in practice?

Chronic renal failure in type 2 diabetes is generally associated with proteinuria when due to diabetic nephropathy. However, there are some patients who have renal impairment but no proteinuria or microalbuminuria. The predominant pathological problem in this group may be glomerulosclerosis. A group in Australia, when reviewing patients with type 2 diabetes and renal impairment (GFR <60 ml/min) attending a specialist renal clinic, found 23% had no proteinuria.[18] These patients were more commonly female and slightly older but the annual rate of decline in GFR was no different from those with proteinuria. Referral for specialist renal advice is appropriate.

Management of these patients is identical to that for patients with proteinuria, with excellent blood pressure control and aggressive treatment of cardiovascular risk factors.

## FUTURE CHANGES

### 14.18 What changes will happen in treatment of diabetic nephropathy?

Improvements in understanding, detection, prevention and intervention for diabetic nephropathy over the past 25 years have been phenomenal as described in previous questions. What has been less successful is the application of the knowledge to the population with type 2 diabetes, with many patients still presenting late with advanced renal disease or failing to understand and adhere to therapy – often too late to allow time for medical therapy to prevent progression to end-stage renal failure.

In the next 10 years, one might hope to see:

- genetic/biochemical tests to detect high-risk individuals
- improved population glycaemic control reducing the incidence
- population-wide application of regular checks for early nephropathy
- wider availability of specialist care, and more joint diabetic–renal care
- evidence-based studies for the best combination anti-hypertensive regimens to prevent progression and reduce coronary heart disease mortality
- improved understanding of the pathophysiology of vascular disease development
- trials showing benefit, or otherwise, of lipid-lowering and other therapies in nephropathy
- improved methods of dialysis, and reduced mortality/morbidity
- improved transplant success, and possibly the growth of kidneys in the laboratory.

**PATIENT QUESTIONS**

**14.19 My doctor says I have diabetic kidney disease, but I feel fine.**

Diabetes does most of its damage quietly without producing pain, discomfort or other symptoms. So it is quite possible to feel perfectly well while damage to your kidneys is taking place. Only at a late stage, when perhaps 80% of function has been lost, do people begin to feel unwell with tiredness, lethargy, nausea, loss of appetite, ankle swelling and itching as common symptoms.

The only way to detect *early* kidney damage is by tests of your blood and urine. This is because the earliest changes show up as minute traces of albumin (a protein) in your urine – this is why most people have regular urine checks (at least once a year).

At a later stage, your blood tests become abnormal and your BP goes up but you will still probably feel no symptoms. Only in the very late stages will you feel unwell and the signs become obvious to you and your doctor: swollen ankles, pale puffy face, high BP.

It is much better to prevent diabetic kidney disease. If caught early, its progress can be substantially slowed or even stopped with better glucose control, BP treatment and other interventions. These are more successful if started early rather than late.

The vital point for prevention is that these regular checks, like the MoT test for cars, are essential if any damage is to be picked up early and appropriate treatment started.

**14.20 If I have got diabetic kidney disease, can you stop my kidneys failing?**

There are now effective treatments available that reduce the rate at which the kidneys deteriorate, and sometimes stop the deterioration altogether. These work best if started early before the kidneys are too badly damaged (*see Q. 14.19*). Particularly important is treatment of blood pressure, but there will be many other aspects of your care to prevent other diabetic complications, and it will be some time before the success of the treatment becomes apparent. You should discuss these with your diabetes and/or kidney specialist.

Should the kidneys eventually fail, there are several methods of what is called 'renal replacement therapy'. These include peritoneal dialysis, haemodialysis (both in hospital and at home) and, sometimes, renal transplantation. The choice of these treatments is a complex issue, not everyone being suitable for each sort, and this again will need to be discussed very carefully with your kidney specialist and his or her team.

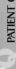 PATIENT QUESTIONS

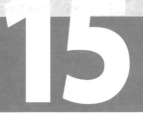

## BACKGROUND TO RETINOPATHY

### 15.1 How can diabetes affect the eye?

The commonest problem is a specific diabetic retinopathy, but there are several other conditions that may occur from the time of presentation onwards (*Box 15.1*).

The refractory changes, often reported at or just after diagnosis, reflect a change in shape of the lens due to the effects of high glucose and resultant osmolarity in increasing its size and thus causing a temporary refractive error. This is sometimes detected first, and diabetes diagnosed, by optometrists – the lens will return to its previous shape and refractive performance after 3–6 weeks of good control; further refraction within that period is unhelpful. These changes often recur with periods of poor control.

Cataract is seen commonly. In older people with type 2 diabetes, the usual senile cataract may be found. When the lens is viewed with an ophthalmoscope, opacities are seen in a spoke fashion around the periphery. Significant cataracts may reduce visual acuity (VA), but also lead to difficulties in screening for diabetic retinopathy as the retinal view is obscured. Referral for assessment and possible lens extraction should be made: most ophthalmologists are happy to proceed to surgery and use a lens implant to maintain good vision.

Occasionally a young person with type 1 diabetes develops a cataract rapidly, often following a period of poor control. In this instance, the lens opacity lies centrally and looks rather like a snowflake when viewed. It is thought the metabolic decompensation causes damage to the lens structure, and that subsequent repair results in this type of cataract.

### CASE VIGNETTE 15.1

A patient with long-standing type 2 diabetes and hypertension but only mild background retinopathy on recent screening has presented with sudden visual loss in her right eye. Is it due to her diabetes?

---

**BOX 15.1  Eye conditions in diabetes**
- Early manifestations:
  - transient refractory changes related to high plasma glucose and osmolarity
  - diabetes cataract
- Late manifestations:
  - diabetic retinopathy and its complications (*see Q. 15.2 onwards*)
  - accelerated senile cataract
  - ocular motor nerve palsies resulting from mononeuritis

---

*Comment*

A sudden vitreous haemorrhage is possible, but very unlikely given her recent screening result. Screening for retinopathy is not 100% effective and, very occasionally, sight-threatening retinopathy is present but not detected. However, if she is hypertensive, it is more probable that she has suffered from a central retinal vein or artery occlusion. The patient requires *urgent* ophthalmological assessment, ideally the same day.

## 15.2 What actually is diabetic retinopathy?

The characteristic changes seen in the retina are known as diabetic retinopathy or diabetic eye disease (*Figs 15.1–15.4*). Features and terms used to describe diabetic retinopathy are outlined in *Table 15.1*.

Chronically high plasma glucose (PG) levels cause damage in the capillary basement membranes and this affects their permeability. Leakage from the capillaries occurs with bleeding and oedema. Capillaries are damaged and then thrombose, leading to ischaemic areas of retina, which in turn respond by producing a number of local growth factors. These stimulate the development of new blood vessels, which may extend unsupported into the vitreous; they are fragile and commonly haemorrhage in the early stages. The new vessels stimulate a significant fibrous tissue response, but the fibrous strands may subsequently contract in time and thus cause retinal detachment.

Proliferative changes are commoner in type 1 diabetes, while macular disease with oedema and exudates is commoner in type 2 diabetes, though

**TABLE 15. 1 Features and terms used to describe diabetic retinopathy**

| Feature/term | Description |
|---|---|
| Dots and blots | Small red lesions due to microaneurysms or small haemorrhages |
| Haemorrhages | Medium or large red areas relating to leakage or bleeding from retinal capillaries or vessels |
| Exudates | Irregular yellow/white lesions with sharp outlines due to the leakage of lipid material from retinal vessels |
| Cotton wool spots | White or grey lesions with indistinct outlines due to the ischaemic retinal areas |
| Venous abnormalities | Include dilated and tortuous irregular veins and arterial changes with irregular vessel diameter and wall sheathing |
| New vessels | Small fine new vessels growing from the retinal veins which later grow to extensive arcades with supporting fibrous tissue |
| Maculopathy | Damage to the macula through oedema or ischaemia |

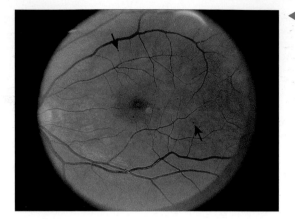

◀ **Fig. 15.1** Minimal diabetic background retinopathy showing only a few microaneurysms (arrows).

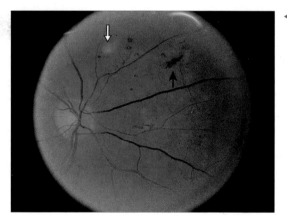

◀ **Fig. 15.2** Moderate diabetic retinopathy showing microaneurysms, haemorrhage (solid arrow) and cotton wool spot (open arrow).

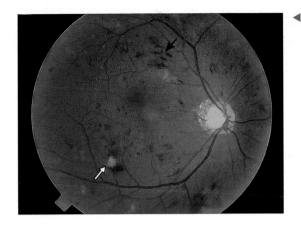

◀ **Fig. 15.3** Extensive diabetic retinopathy showing multiple microaneurysms, haemorrhages (solid arrow) and cotton wool spots (open arrow).

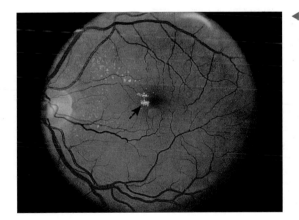

◀ **Fig. 15.4** Sight-threatening maculopathy due to diabetic retinopathy showing exudates in the macula area (arrow)

some patients will develop both features. This difference is probably due to age-related changes in the vitreous rather than to the type of diabetes. Since the macula has the highest acuity of the whole retina, any damage to it will impair VA.

### 15.3 How likely are people with diabetes to get diabetic retinopathy?

Diabetic retinopathy remains the commonest cause of blindness in the working age population in the UK and most Western countries, with a blindness incidence of about 60 per 100 000 patients per year.

Significant damage is not, however, an inevitable consequence of diabetes. The prevalence of retinopathy is related to duration of disease and glycaemic control. While the annual *incidence* is relatively low, the cumulative *prevalence* of retinopathy is high, especially detected with sensitive modern techniques.[1] Most people with type 1 diabetes will develop at least some features of retinopathy after 20–30 years of diabetes but a much smaller proportion will have sight-threatening eye disease (STED), the really worrying stage.[2]

Between 10 and 40% of patients with type 2 diabetes have some degree of retinopathy *at the time of diagnosis*, with a small number having STED.[3]

*Figure 15.5* shows the relationship between control and proliferative retinopathy for type 1 diabetes.

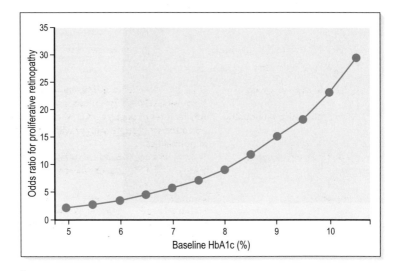

**Fig. 15.5** The relationship between baseline HbA1c and odds ratio for progression to proliferative retinopathy from the EURODIAB study of type 1 diabetes. Note the extreme risk variation between HbA1c of <6 and >10%. (From Porta et al.[6] Copyright © 2001 Springer Verlag.)

### 15.4 What is meant by 'background' retinopathy?

A classification and scoring system for diabetic retinopathy has been established which helps in managing patients and predicting prognosis[4] (*Table 15.2*).

Background retinopathy describes the earliest changes seen in diabetes: it does not usually cause visual loss unless the macula area is involved. The dots, blots, exudates and haemorrhages seen in background retinopathy are not permanent features; serial photographs show that individual lesions disappear with haemorrhages being absorbed, but with new lesions frequently developing. Not all patients with background retinopathy will progress to more serious sight-threatening problems, but all patients must be regularly monitored to detect those progressing to STED.

Patients with pre-proliferative retinopathy are at high risk of developing new vessels that potentially can cause visual loss. They need regular review by an ophthalmologist with special expertise in diabetic eye disease. If close follow-up is difficult and progression is likely due to other risk factors such as renal failure or hypertension, it may be preferable to undertake laser treatment *before* new vessels occur – fluorescein angiography of the retina is helpful in clarifying the extent of disease.

**TABLE 15.2  A simple classification of diabetic retinopathy**

| Type of retinopathy | Description |
| --- | --- |
| Background retinopathy | Dots, blots, exudates and haemorrhages may be present with <6 cotton wool spots |
| Pre-proliferative retinopathy | Any features of background retinopathy with ≥6 cotton wool spots, with or without venous abnormalities |
| Proliferative retinopathy | New vessels developing either from the disc and/or the peripheral retina with or without fibrous proliferation |
| Maculopathy | Damage to the macula area due to oedema commonly associated with exudates at the macula, or due to ischaemia with extensive capillary closure in the macula area |

## RISK AND SCREENING

### 15.5 How can patients reduce the risk of developing diabetic eye disease?

Known risk factors affecting development or progression of retinopathy are:[5]
- existing retinopathy, and increasing microaneurysm count
- poor glycaemic control: some studies suggest >10-fold increase in risk for HbA1c of 10% versus 6%[6]
- raised blood pressure
- long duration of diabetes
- presence of proteinuria or microalbuminuria
- dyslipidaemia
- anaemia
- pregnancy.

The most effective way of preventing serious retinopathy is to achieve and maintain excellent glycaemic control (*see Case vignette 15.2*). This was demonstrated for type 1 diabetes in the DCCT where there was a substantial reduction in development or progression of retinopathy by 54–76% for different measures.[7]

In type 2 diabetes, most people have had a long period of unrecognised hyperglycaemia, which results in a significant proportion having retinopathy at the time of diagnosis (*see Q. 15.3*). The UKPDS showed useful reductions for first laser treatment and cataract extraction from improved control (*Table 15.3*).[8]

Blood pressure is also important. Again UKPDS data (*Fig. 15.6, see also Fig. 2.4B*) show a clear relationship between increased BP and the risk of developing diabetic retinopathy; intensive BP treatment substantially reduced both the risk of retinopathy and its progression.[9]

Aspirin has been shown to have no beneficial effect on diabetic eye disease.[10]

---

**TABLE 15.3  The development of retinopathy in UKPDS comparing intensive blood glucose control with conventional control in people with type 2 diabetes**

|  | Conventional therapy | Intensive therapy | Relative risk reduction |
|---|---|---|---|
| First laser treatment | 1.1 | 0.79 | 29%, p = 0.003 |
| Vitreous haemorrhage | 0.09 | 0.07 | 23%, p = NS |
| Blind in one eye | 0.35 | 0.29 | 16%, p = NS |
| Cataract extraction | 0.74 | 0.56 | 24%, p <0.05 |

All rates are per 100 patient-years. NS, not significant.

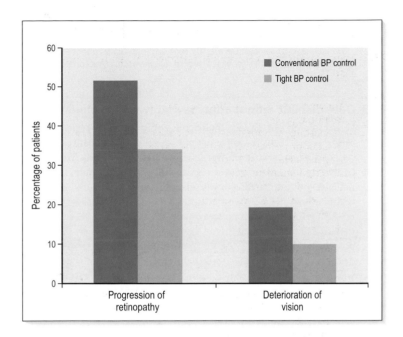

**Fig. 15.6** The progression of retinopathy according to tight or conventional control of BP after 7.5 years' follow-up in UKPDS (drawn from data in UK Prospective Diabetes Study Group[9]).

## CASE VIGNETTE 15.2

A 65-year-old man with type 2 diabetes for 7 years already has moderate background retinopathy and is seen 6-monthly in the ophthalmology clinic. His BP is 152/94 mmHg and BMI 32 kg/m$^2$. Current drugs include metformin 500 mg twice daily, ramipril 10 mg daily, simvastatin 40 mg daily and aspirin 75 mg daily. Current results are: HbA1c 8.1%, creatinine 76 µmol/l, albumin:creatinine ratio 1.8 mg/mmol. What else can be done?

*Comment*

His glycaemic control is not ideal and needs to be improved, aiming to reduce HbA1c to normal if possible. The UKPDS showed that patients with HbA1c in the lowest tertile (<6.2%) had the smallest risk of retinopathy progression. The first step would be to increase the metformin dose but then to consider the addition of a sulphonylurea or 'glitazone' if control is still not ideal.

Blood pressure control is also poor. In patients with retinopathy, the target is to maintain BP at 130/80 mmHg or less. The intensive BP treatment arm of the UKPDS showed a 35% reduction in the risk of laser photocoagulation. The next step should probably include a low-dose diuretic, for example bendroflumethiazide (bendrofluazide) 2.5 mg daily or, if not suitable, a beta-blocker such as atenolol 50 mg daily or a calcium antagonist such as felodipine 5–10 mg daily. Many patients require three or four drugs to control BP adequately.

He will need to be seen frequently for a while to achieve these targets, which will also benefit other microvascular and macrovascular outcomes.

## 15.6 Does diabetic retinopathy inevitably lead to blindness?

No, absolutely not. In fact, the lesions come and go, especially in the earlier stages. However, once patients develop maculopathy or proliferative retinopathy, progression towards visual loss is eventually likely unless treated. In the American Wisconsin epidemiological study, 24% of patients with untreated eyes with proliferative retinopathy were blind within 4 years.[2,3] Laser photocoagulation reduces the risk of blindness by 60–80% compared with no treatment. It is most effective if used before there is significant visual loss. A few patients do, however, show rapidly progressive disease and, despite treatment, lose vision. Once STED develops, prompt specialist ophthalmologist assessment is necessary, with no delay in photocoagulation if indicated. Laser treatment for macular disease is effective, but to a lesser extent than for proliferative disease.

## 15.7 Why is screening necessary to detect diabetic eye disease?

Diabetic retinopathy is nearly always asymptomatic until quite serious. Deterioration in vision (reported by the patient or a measured drop in VA) is a *late* feature; *the only early clues come from retinal examination.*

Thus someone with serious proliferative retinopathy can be entirely unaware of the condition until they have a vitreous haemorrhage. They then notice a sudden deterioration in vision but the retina is difficult to examine as blood in the vitreous obscures the view. Laser photocoagulation to shrink the new vessels may not be possible until the haemorrhage is reabsorbed which usually takes 4–6 weeks. If further bleeding occurs, treatment is delayed. Fibrous proliferation begins to occur and can lead to permanent visual loss through retinal detachment.

In maculopathy, vision is usually affected at an earlier stage but laser treatment is unable to restore vision to normal. Laser photocoagulation retards the progression rather than restoring vision, and so works best if undertaken before there is a significant reduction in VA.

It remains extremely disappointing that, when trials over 20 years ago demonstrated the efficacy of photocoagulation in reducing blindness, screening for diabetic eye disease is still patchy. In most countries there is, as yet, no convincing evidence of a reduction in the incidence of visual loss from diabetes.

## 15.8 Is measuring visual acuity an adequate check?

No, definitely not (*see Q. 15.7*). Since visual deterioration is a late feature of retinopathy, normal distant VA does not exclude significant retinal damage. In contrast, reduced corrected VA is an indication for immediate investigation/referral as it indicates reduced vision, though not necessarily related to diabetes.

## 15.9 What is the best method to use for screening?

The National Screening Committee in the UK, and most other international authorities, have recommended using digital retinal photography to screen for diabetic retinopathy. This represents the 'gold standard' because of its high sensitivity in detecting retinopathy and the ease of quality assurance as a permanent image is created.[11,12]

Distant corrected VA is measured for each eye. This is undertaken using a standard chart (e.g. Snellen chart) at a fixed distance. Best achieved VA is recorded by asking the patient to use their glasses, or a pinhole which can correct for refractive error.

A high-quality digital image is then taken, usually through dilated pupils. The image is reviewed by a trained retinal grader, who refers patients with sight-threatening or significant retinopathy to an ophthalmologist. In patients with dense lens opacities, it may be impossible to obtain a suitable retinal image and these patients may need to be examined by indirect ophthalmoscopy.

Digital retinal photography is initially expensive because of the capital equipment costs. Some areas still rely on retinal photographs using a conventional camera to screen. In other areas, screening programmes have utilised trained optometrists who work in optician practices in the community. These programmes may have a lower sensitivity in detecting retinopathy but may reach a higher proportion of the population at risk, as they are easier to access in the community. Many rural communities have travelling cameras to increase accessibility and images can be read electronically at a distance; indeed automated readers can now detect some, but not all, lesions.

Several studies have shown that persistent non-attenders have worse outcomes for retinopathy and other complications.

### 15.10 When and how often should people with diabetes be screened for retinopathy?

The current UK and US recommendation is to screen all people with type 2 diabetes annually from diagnosis, and for type 1 diabetes to screen annually after 5 years' duration. Other countries (New Zealand, Australia) recommend every 2 years for low-risk individuals, more often for high-risk and starting after 3–4 years' duration for type 1 diabetes.

There has been some analysis of retinopathy risk in people with no detectable disease to attempt to reduce the screening frequency and to tailor it more accurately for those at higher risk.[13] The UKPDS suggests that those at low risk could be screened every 2–3 years: this has been strengthened by a recent Liverpool study.[14]

At present, there remains considerable anxiety about implementing this policy, as concern about missing treatable retinopathy is a real worry. Patients in the UKPDS may not be typical of those with diabetes in the real world!

It also appears that some high-risk individuals may need to be reviewed more frequently than annually.

The following patient characteristics increase the risk of retinopathy developing or progressing and such individuals should be screened *at least* annually:

- ■ Known diabetes duration >10 years
- ■ Patients on insulin rather than diet or oral agents
- ■ Those with chronic poor glycaemic control
- ■ Those with hypertension and/or nephropathy
- ■ Those with even trivial lesions near the macula.

## ISSUES WITH PROVEN DIABETIC RETINOPATHY

### 15.11 Do all patients with diabetic eye disease need to see an ophthalmologist?

No. Those with minimal or mild background retinopathy with no involvement of the macula area do not need to see an ophthalmologist, but do require regular monitoring (annually or more often, *see Q. 15.10*) to detect progression to STED. These patients can usually be monitored either by retinal photography or, alternatively, by fundoscopy by an experienced diabetologist. In some areas, the ophthalmologist will undertake this monitoring process but it is critical that the routine workload related to monitoring minor disease does not prevent rapid access for people with sight-threatening problems.

Once retinopathy progresses to pre-proliferative or proliferative retinopathy, or if maculopathy is present, regular follow-up by an ophthalmologist is vital. Close liaison with the diabetologist is important and many departments operate a joint diabetic–eye clinic with both specialists present.

Patients with sudden visual loss should be seen within 24 hours, those with vitreous haemorrhage or new vessels within a week and those with unexplained visual acuity loss or macular oedema within 4 weeks.

## 15.12 What happens when retinopathy is identified for the first time?

The first step is to explain the finding to the patient. It should not be dismissed as trivial, even if it is only a few microaneurysms. Many are devastated by the development of a 'complication'; they had come to terms with their diabetes and learnt how to cope with the day-to-day treatment. The new diagnosis often leads to a resurgence of all those initial worries about the seriousness of the disease. One can liken it to the patient with treated cancer who finds they now have a metastasis. Being sympathetic but reassuring is vital and it is helpful to show them their retinal photograph or a similar one to explain the changes, especially what 'mild' and 'moderate' etc. mean.

Next it is vital to stress the positive treatment options of reducing the progression of retinopathy by improving glycaemic control where possible and maintaining normal BP levels.[7–9] Patients with retinopathy should aim to keep their BP at 130/80 mmHg or less (*see Ch. 13*).

## 15.13 Is it true that improving glycaemic control can lead to worsening of retinopathy?

Yes, in the short term, but not that often.[15] In several studies that produced rapid improvement in glycaemic control (often using insulin pumps), a few patients showed a transient worsening of retinopathy for up to 12–18 months. However, when the cases were reviewed after 2–3 years, the long-term visual outcome was improved, i.e. the short-term deterioration was more than balanced by the longer-term benefit. In the first year of the DCCT, significant deterioration occurred in 2% of conventionally treated patients in whom glycaemic control did not change compared with 5% of intensively treated patients who on average lowered their HbA1c by 2%.

Deterioration in retinopathy is probably related to reduced retinal blood flow. Since hyperglycaemia is associated with increased capillary flow, normalising PG levels can lead to a small reduction in blood flow that, in ischaemic areas of the retina, may be critical and cause retinal infarcts to appear. These in turn stimulate new blood vessel formation. Most of these cases showed progression to pre-proliferative retinopathy.

In those with very poor glycaemic control and florid background or pre-proliferative retinopathy, it is sensible to improve glycaemic control gradually over a period of months rather than weeks. The retinopathy may need to be reviewed more frequently than usual, and laser treatment possibly undertaken earlier rather than later. Diabetic retinopathy is also seen in pregnancy.

## LASER AND OTHER TREATMENTS

### 15.14 What treatment is available for diabetic retinopathy?

The mainstay of treatment is laser photocoagulation which aims to stabilise the retina and prevent progression of the disease.[16,17] In maculopathy (the commonest lesion in type 2 diabetes), the small capillaries in the macula area become leaky and oedema develops. This distorts the fovea and so vision is affected. A characteristic feature is circinate exudates, with the leaking capillaries in the centre. Laser photocoagulation is undertaken to seal the leaking capillaries by applying a number of small burns. Obviously, photocoagulation must avoid the fovea and its immediate surroundings otherwise permanent visual impairment will result. If it is not clear where the leaking capillaries are sited and there is significant macular oedema, laser treatment is undertaken in a grid fashion.

Patients with maculopathy are usually treated as outpatients and it takes only a few minutes to perform the treatment. The laser is connected to the slit lamp and operated by the ophthalmologist as the retina is viewed. The treatment itself is painless. Patients with maculopathy may require laser treatment on several occasions as fresh lesions appear, suggesting persistent capillary leakage. Generally, patients are reviewed at 3–6-monthly intervals.

Patients with proliferative retinopathy are also treated with laser photocoagulation but the aim of treatment is different. The stimulus to the development of new vessels is thought to be areas of ischaemia in the peripheral retina. Laser photocoagulation is not aimed at the new vessels themselves – instead, burns are made throughout the peripheral retina avoiding only the macula area. The goal is to destroy the ischaemic areas but leave some remaining normal tissue between burns. Frequently, hundreds of small burns are made which takes a considerable time: this is called pan-retinal ablation.

On the first occasion, the photocoagulation is not usually painful but often more than one treatment session is needed and the retina seems to become sensitised to the treatment with resulting discomfort, requiring local anaesthetic or, rarely, a full general anaesthetic.

## 15.15 Does photocoagulation have side effects?

 Focal laser treatment for maculopathy does not usually cause any major problem for most patients, though few enjoy the experience. Some will notice a transient change in their VA but it should settle within a few days. Patients treated with a pan-retinal ablation may notice a change in their vision. Generally, the distant VA is maintained but some describe a change in the quality of images perceived.

Destruction of a significant amount of peripheral retina causes problems with night vision, sensitivity to high intensity sunlight and a reduction in peripheral vision. Formal testing of visual fields can highlight significant field restriction after pan-retinal photocoagulation. These problems can lead to difficulty with driving. In the UK, the DVLA has strict regulations relating to driving; all patients having laser treatment for retinopathy must undergo formal field testing and examination by an ophthalmologist or optometrist (*see also Q. 11.14*).

Many patients with retinopathy appear to go through a few years when the eye disease is active and progressive. If vision is preserved during this time by laser photocoagulation, the retinopathy often then becomes quiescent and remains so for the rest of their lives. Thus, one sees many patients who were successfully treated for proliferative retinopathy or maculopathy in the past.

## 15.16 What if laser treatment is unsuccessful?

A proportion of patients with vitreous haemorrhage, fibrovascular proliferation and diffuse macular oedema will benefit from vitrectomy. This is a specialist ophthalmologist decision.

Despite optimal treatment, a small number of patients will lose their sight. Expert community support involving the Royal National Institute for the Blind or similar organisations, together with low vision aids should be provided.

## 15.17 Which conditions can lead to more rapid progression of retinopathy?

Certain groups of patients seem to have more rapidly progressive retinopathy, of which important factors include chronic renal failure, nephrotic syndrome, uncontrolled hypertension, pregnancy and prolonged very poor glycaemic control.

These patients may need to be more closely supervised by an ophthalmologist. It is imperative the ophthalmologist is made aware of the risk factors involved, and that all members of the team work together.

### 15.18 Which patients get proliferative retinopathy and maculopathy, and can patients have both?

In general, people with type 1 diabetes tend to develop proliferative retinopathy, whilst those with type 2 more commonly have maculopathy (*see Q. 15.14*) However, both conditions are seen in both groups of patients. A few unfortunate individuals do have both types of retinopathy at the same time. In some patients with proliferative retinopathy, the maculopathy is due to retinal ischaemia which is not treatable by photocoagulation.

### 15.19 What other treatments may become available for retinopathy?

There are several possible advances already in trials:

- Trials of angiotensin converting enzyme inhibitors and angiotensin 2 blockers are underway.[18]
- Increased low density lipoprotein cholesterol is recognised to be a risk factor for proliferative retinopathy and maculopathy. Several trials of statins are in progress, especially ASPEN using atorvastatin.
- A new protein kinase C inhibitor is being used but initial results are not as promising as had been expected.
- Studies using octreotide or similar agents that are potent inhibitors of growth hormone release.

Other expected advances in this area include automated computer reading of retinal photographs, and more precise targeting of retinal screening so that screening frequency will match the risk.

 **PATIENT QUESTION**

#### 15.20 Can I drive after having drops at my annual eye examination?

Drops are put in the eye before screening to dilate your pupils. The drops can affect your ability to focus properly, particularly if you try to read or do close work. In bright sunlight, the pupils usually become small to prevent dazzle. The drops prevent this happening, and so you may not see entirely normally and/or be dazzled by sunlight or headlights. People are therefore advised not to drive for about 2–3 hours afterwards.

PATIENT QUESTIONS

# Neuropathy

# 16

## BACKGROUND TO NEUROPATHY

### 16.1 What are the different types of neuropathy seen in diabetes?

Diabetic neuropathy can affect any nerve in the body, but there are a number of common clinical pictures[1] which include:

- peripheral neuropathy affecting predominantly the sensation of the feet and legs in a symmetrical pattern – the 'glove and stocking' distribution
- 'femoral amyotrophy' affecting one or both thighs with a large motor component
- focal vascular neuropathy involving single nerves, of which diplopia as a consequence of third or sixth cranial nerve involvement is commonest
- autonomic neuropathy.

### 16.2 How common is diabetic neuropathy?

Surprisingly common. One community study found that 16% of people with diabetes had evidence of neuropathy compared with 3% of people without diabetes.[2] In this study, 17% of patients with type 2 diabetes had neuropathy compared with 13% of those with type 1 diabetes, though this will depend very substantially on the duration of diabetes (*Fig. 16.1*). Chronic neuropathy is rare before 5 years' duration of type 1 diabetes, though it is often present at the time of diagnosis in type 2 disease.[3]

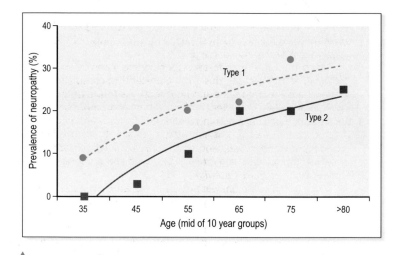

**Fig. 16.1** The prevalence of peripheral neuropathy in type 1 and type 2 diabetes related to age, with the trend lines for each group.

The prevalence also increases with age, greater height, increasing alcohol intake, and poorer control as judged by HbA1c;[4] it is commonly associated with retinopathy and with nephropathy.

### 16.3 What causes diabetic neuropathy?

Neuropathy is due to damage to the nerves resulting in abnormal function. The mechanism of damage is not completely understood, with metabolic and vascular theories competing – though both may be relevant.[1,5] Hyperglycaemia at an intracellular level leads to abnormal function, which may be associated with increased excitability of the nerves and increased conduction of impulses causing hyperaesthesia. Longer-term damage may also be related to metabolic or vascular effects. The capillaries supplying peripheral nerves can become leaky and damaged as is seen in other microvascular complications. Ultimately capillary closure occurs with resulting ischaemia to the nerve cells. It is interesting that the longest nerves of the body – those supplying the feet – are the most severely damaged. Also, taller and older people have a higher incidence of neuropathy, presumably as their longer nerves are more vulnerable to the damaging effects of hyperglycaemia.

## PRESENTATION AND DIAGNOSIS

### 16.4 What are the common presentations of peripheral neuropathy?

Patients with peripheral neuropathy most often present with numbness and/or paraesthesia, pain, foot ulceration or muscle weakness due to nerve damage.

The commonest manifestation is numbness and/or paraesthesia. However, in many cases, this is not a presenting complaint as patients are asymptomatic and neuropathy is found only on direct questioning. Pain in the feet is also relatively common: patients describe the pain as a burning feeling or like 'pins and needles'. Typically it is at its worst at night, often leading to loss of sleep. It is often aggravated by heat and/or pressure (e.g. of bedclothes) and relieved by cold. The pain is difficult to treat and responds poorly to normal analgesia (see Case vignette 16.1).

Many patients are unaware of the onset and progression of neuropathy as it is frequently painless. Their first presentation with a foot ulcer often results from damage to the foot due to a shoe rubbing or standing on an unperceived sharp object. Despite significant trauma, the patient may feel little or no pain and may be unaware of the lesion, often continuing to walk with little discomfort and only presenting late when spreading infection has developed from the initial break in the skin.

■ *Amyotrophy or femoral neuropathy*: Less commonly the patient may present with muscle weakness due to neuropathy. In the case of 'amyotrophy', weakness in the thigh muscles develops gradually over a period of a few weeks, usually accompanied by severe pain. It can be asymmetrical (affecting one thigh only) or bilateral (usually more severe in one leg than the other).

■ *Mononeuropathies*: The sudden onset of diplopia, due to weakness in the eye muscle, is caused by damage to one of the third or sixth ocular nerves. This is thought to be due to sudden occlusion of the vasa vasorum. This can happen to any nerve and usually recovery occurs over a period of weeks. Other nerves that may be involved include the facial nerve (Bell's palsy), the lateral cutaneous nerve of the thigh and also intercostal nerves. Unusual manifestations should prompt referral to a specialist.

## 16.5  How do I diagnose diabetic neuropathy?

The most important first step in diagnosing diabetic neuropathy is to have a high index of suspicion – but always be prepared to exclude other possible

---

**BOX 16.1  Important differential diagnoses of diabetic neuropathy**

■ Distal symmetrical neuropathy:
— vitamin B12 or folate deficiency
— hypothyroidism
— uraemia
— alcohol
■ Autonomic neuropathy:
— Shy–Drager syndrome (progressive autonomic failure)
— idiopathic orthostatic hypotension
■ Diffuse motor neuropathy:
— Guillain–Barré syndrome
— myasthenia gravis
■ Femoral neuropathy:
— degenerative spinal disc disease
— intrinsic spinal cord mass lesion
— cauda equina lesion
■ Cranial neuropathy:
— carotid aneurysm
— intracranial mass
■ Mononeuritis multiplex:
— vasculitis
— neurosyphilis
— amyloid

causes of neurological problems (*see Case vignette 16.2 and Box 16.1*). The classic symptoms are given above (*see Q. 16.4*).

Affected nerves may be in any area of the body and can also seem to move from one area to another over a period of weeks. The character and site of the discomfort need to be carefully documented, and relieving or precipitating factors explored. In general, exercise does not exacerbate pain in neuropathy and probably most characteristic is the severity at night. If nocturnal exacerbation is absent, it is unlikely to be due to diabetic neuropathy.

Many other patients will have no symptoms and neuropathy will only be identified on direct questioning and/or examination. A careful history is important to consider other possible causes of neuropathy and to look for supporting features. Alcohol intake and smoking history are important, as are enquiries about erectile function in men.

Neurological examination should include testing for tone, muscle power and reflexes. Sensory testing should include light touch, pinprick discrimination, proprioception and vibration perception. Stroking the skin with a tissue and asking the patient to tell you where the sensation is increased is useful for identifying areas of hyperaesthesia. This needs to be done with care, as it may be quite uncomfortable for the patient. Patients with significant suspected neuropathy should be referred to a diabetic specialist and/or podiatrist for assessment, investigation and further management.

## 16.6 Does alcohol intake affect painful neuropathy?

There is little hard evidence on this issue, but clinical anecdote strongly suggests that heavy alcohol intake, or a history of alcohol-related problems, can produce more severe pain than would be expected from the diabetic neuropathy alone.

## 16.7 How do you screen for neuropathy?

Screening for diabetic neuropathy should be one of the annual review checks.[6] A full neurological examination is unnecessary when screening. The patient should be instructed to remove their shoes and socks, and the feet examined for any ulcers, deformity or build-up of callus. It is important to diagnose asymptomatic neuropathy as the patient needs education about avoiding diabetic foot disease.

The easiest screening test for neuropathy is to use a 10G monofilament on six places on each foot (after callus has been removed) as shown in *Figure 16.2*. The monofilament is a fine plastic stick, the tip of which is applied to the skin with sufficient pressure to bend it slightly – the patient (with their eyes closed) is asked if they can feel it. If the patient is unable to feel fewer than four out of six places in either foot, then neuropathy is present. If a monofilament is unavailable, then a piece of cotton wool can

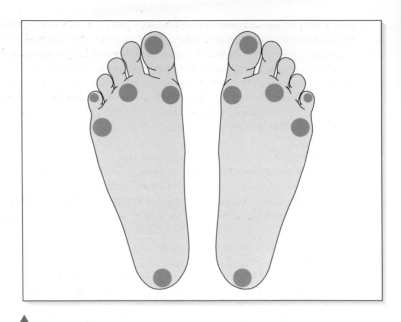

**Fig. 16.2** Recommended filament testing sites, after callus has been removed. (From New Zealand Guidelines Group. Available online at *www.nzgg.org.nz.*)

be used to check light touch sensation at six places over each foot. If sensory abnormalities are found a fuller neurological examination should be undertaken to define its extent. Ankle reflexes are usually absent and, in more severe cases, knee reflexes also. Loss of vibration sensation is found at an early stage with lack of pinpoint discrimination and impaired proprioception as it progresses.

Some patients present with typical symptoms of neuropathy but when examined have completely normal sensation. They are still likely to have significant neuropathy, the clinical tests being relatively insensitive, and the nerve function, although disturbed, is still reasonably preserved. If you are unsure, specialist nerve conduction studies can be helpful. The prognosis for recovery and outcome is good in these patients.

## TREATMENT

### 16.8 What is the optimal treatment for painful neuropathy?

Neuropathic pain can be difficult to treat because the pain responds poorly to normal analgesia.[6,7] Patients often get severely depressed and frequently lose weight. In most cases of 'diabetic amyotrophy', the painful symptoms will improve with time but this may take 9–18 months. An explanation to the patient of the problem and reassurance that, in the long term, the pain will disappear is important. Pain resolves as either the nerves recover normal function or the nerve damage progresses and pain perception is lost altogether. Providing support and reassurance through this difficult time is crucial. Sometimes it is valuable for a patient to talk to someone who has suffered a similar problem.

### Glycaemic control

Improving glycaemic control is the only treatment that has been shown to shorten the duration or extent of symptoms other than pain. This means achieving glycaemic control, with HbA1c in the normal range if possible. For many patients with type 2 diabetes, this requires conversion to insulin therapy.

### Control of pain

Control of the painful symptoms needs to be tackled logically and progressively. A clear explanation of the aims of treatment will help the patient to understand the likely benefits.

Paracetamol before bed may help patients with mild symptoms. It is generally not possible to achieve freedom from pain, but tricyclic antidepressants remain the first line of treatment as they also promote sleep and raise the pain threshold. In one trial of gabapentin, 60% of patients had a moderate improvement in pain scores but only a few were free from pain.[8] Treatment is aimed at controlling the pain by making it more bearable and promoting sleep at night, thus early use of agents to raise the pain threshold is valuable. But it is also helpful to provide potent analgesia with opiates for crises or difficult times in the day. Rarely pain clinic advice may need to be sought.

### Management of pain in neuropathy

- Try simple analgesics (e.g. paracetamol or ibuprofen), taken *before* bedtime.
- Use physical treatments such as wearing socks or tights in bed at night to prevent bedclothes touching skin, try rubbing in creams such as capsaicin 0.075% or occlusive dressings such as Op-site. Isosorbide dinitrate spray has recently been shown to be beneficial.
- Start amitriptyline 25 mg 1–2 hrs before bed to act by raising the pain threshold – increase to 75–150 mg if required. It can be used in combination with ordinary analgesics. It will take 2–3 weeks to have maximal effect. Watch out for worsening postural hypotension if the patient has autonomic neuropathy.

■ Try gabapentin, an anticonvulsant, if amitriptyline is unhelpful. Start with 300 mg daily and increase to 600 mg three times daily over 2 weeks. It will be clear within 2 weeks of the full dose whether it has been helpful. If there is no improvement then withdraw slowly over a week as sudden withdrawal can lead to convulsions. Other anticonvulsants (carbamazepine or sodium valproate) have been used in this situation but gabapentin appears to be the most helpful. All these drugs work by raising the pain threshold and making pain more tolerable: patients still need conventional analgesia as well.

■ Use opiates as a last resort if pain is still uncontrolled. Long-acting morphine preparations (e.g. MST, tramadol) are valuable and of proven benefit at night. Recognise the patient who is desperate because of lack of sleep and prescribe opiates for a short spell to allow the patient to get some rest.

## 16.9 Does neuropathy get better?

Some patients appear to develop painful neuropathy following a period of poor control, or soon after diagnosis in type 2 diabetes (*Case vignette 16.1*). By the time there are symptoms, glycaemic control is often good: one speculation is that a relatively acute deterioration in nerve function follows either a period of poor control or sudden improvement. In these cases, it is not uncommon to find quite severe pain with little objective evidence of damage. Recovery is the usual outcome but it may take a period of months.

Those who present with amyotrophy generally make a reasonable recovery but this usually takes 9–18 months. Most patients with mononeuropathies such as third or sixth nerve palsies recover over a period of 6–12 weeks.

In patients with insensate neuropathy, the onset is often more insidious and significant recovery is unlikely. The patient is usually left with numb, insensitive feet which are at high risk of diabetic foot disease, though the lack of discomfort may mislead them. Education about suitable footwear and regular examination of the feet are vital so that prevention or early recognition of a potential problem occurs. These patients need rapid direct access to a specialist diabetic foot service when problems develop.[9]

**CASE VIGNETTE 16.1**

An elderly patient is complaining of severe burning pain in both feet for the last 3 weeks. It keeps him awake at night and has not responded to paracetamol. He was diagnosed with type 2 diabetes 3 months ago, and had been making excellent progress. At diagnosis, his fasting glucose was 15.2 mmol/l and HbA1c 11.5% but with a careful diet, he has lost 5 kg in weight. At his last visit 2 months after diagnosis, metformin 500 mg twice daily was commenced, as HbA1c was 8.5%. How do you manage his new problem?

*Comment*

A full history needs to be taken to identify any precipitating or relieving factors. Bedclothes touching the skin at night and waking the patient from sleep often aggravate the burning pain. The pain, although present during the day, is usually less problematic than at night. Once awake patients find it impossible to get back to sleep: hanging the foot out of bed to cool it is classical and would confirm this. However, pain worsened by exercise is more likely to be due to peripheral arterial disease or arthritis. Patients also describe severe lancing-type pain that may last only a few seconds.

Alcohol and smoking history should be reviewed – often previous or current excessive alcohol appears to exacerbate the pain

Examination should be undertaken, testing tone, power and reflexes in the legs. Sensation should be tested for light touch, pinprick discrimination, vibration perception and proprioception. Initial (and possibly specialist) investigations (*Box 16.2*) should be undertaken, as well as reassessment of current glycaemic control with fasting blood glucose (BG) and HbA1c.

He is probably suffering from an acute sensory neuropathy related to the rapid change in control from poor control at diagnosis to the marked improvement within 2 months. A clear explanation is required with the assurance that this will improve but it will take time for the nerves to recover.

Achieving excellent control should be possible by increasing the dose of metformin if HbA1c is still >6.5% and, if this is inadequate, adding a sulphonylurea or glitazone. Commencing amitriptyline at night and trying a stronger analgesic such as co-dydramol would be the first step in trying to control his symptoms. If increasing doses of amitriptyline failed to improve his symptoms, a switch to gabapentin would be the next step. At this stage he may need the help of opiates to gain some pain relief. During the next 6–18 months he will require considerable support and reassurance that the pain will disappear with time.

---

### BOX 16.2 Investigations for patients with suspected neuropathy

- ■ Initial:
  - — haemoglobin and ESR
  - — urea and electrolytes, serum creatinine
  - — thyroid function test
  - — liver function tests including gamma glutamyl-transpeptidase (GGT)
  - — venereal diseases research laboratory test (VDRL)
  - — antinuclear antibodies
- ■ Further specialist investigations according to patient symptoms and signs:
  - — nerve conduction studies
  - — MRI of spine
  - — CT of brain

## AUTONOMIC NEUROPATHY

### 16.10 What is autonomic neuropathy and how does it present?

This involves nerve damage to the sympathetic and parasympathetic nervous systems. Most patients with autonomic problems will already have evidence of a distal peripheral neuropathy and often either retinopathy or nephropathy (or both). It is generally seen in patients with type 1 diabetes of long duration.[10]

Patients can present with a variety of symptoms affecting several different systems (*Box 16.3*) or they be completely unaware of the problem.

### 16.11 What are the specific systems involved by autonomic neuropathy?

*Cardiovascular system*

Cardiovascular symptoms can include devastating postural hypotension so that each time the patient tries to stand up they feel very light headed due to low BP. A drop of ≥30 mmHg in systolic BP after 2 or more minutes' standing is characteristic. Falls are frequent. Investigation and treatment are needed, the latter to include avoiding all drugs that aggravate the problem. Some patients respond to elastic stockings or fludrocortisone, but the latter must be used carefully as it can cause fluid retention and heart failure. Specialist assessment is advised for any patient with major autonomic neuropathy.

---

**BOX 16.3  Common types of autonomic neuropathy**

- Cardiovascular:
  — postural hypotension
  — persistent tachycardia due to parasympathetic damage
  — cardiac dysrhythmias
- Gastrointestinal:
  — gastroparesis with vomiting and delayed stomach emptying
  — gustatory sweating (pronounced sweating after eating)
  — colonic dysfunction with diarrhoea and incontinence or constipation
- Genitourinary:
  — sexual dysfunction including impotence
  — bladder dysfunction including retention

---

### Gastrointestinal system

Gastrointestinal presentations may include repeated episodes of unprovoked vomiting associated with nausea, and often with unstable glycaemic control. It is seen most commonly in patients with type 1 diabetes and again there are usually other significant microvascular complications. It is important to take a thorough history, complete a full examination and investigate to exclude other pathology such as peptic ulceration or stricture. Delayed gastric emptying can be demonstrated with radioisotope studies. Endoscopy is valuable to exclude other treatable causes of vomiting such as gastritis, peptic ulceration or stricture. Unfortunately, this often responds poorly to treatment but simple anti-emetics such as metoclopramide should be tried. Domperidone can sometimes be quite valuable but referral is advised. Varying absorption of food as gastric emptying is delayed or food is vomited leads to erratic glycaemic control. Switching to multiple injections of short-acting insulin with long-acting insulin once or twice daily is usually needed to manage the alarming swings in glucose levels.

Excessive sweating after eating (gustatory sweating) is a rare form of autonomic neuropathy (*see Case vignette 16.2*).

Episodes of diarrhoea, especially at night, are another symptom of autonomic neuropathy when it affects the colon. The bowel movements can be very precipitant leading to faecal incontinence in some. Other pathology should be excluded by a full history, examination and appropriate investigations. Treatment is usually with constipating agents such as codeine or loperamide and avoiding dietary precipitants. Occasionally and anecdotally, it responds to oral tetracycline.

### Genitourinary system

Erectile dysfunction or impotence, which affects people with both type 1 and type 2 diabetes, is probably the commonest manifestation of autonomic neuropathy. It can be difficult to discover whether this is due solely to neuropathy or whether there is a significant component due to peripheral vascular disease (*see Qs 12.20–12.24*).

## CASE VIGNETTE 16.2

A middle-aged patient with type 1 diabetes complains of sudden, severe episodes of facial sweating for the last 2 months. He describes episodes of drenching sweats whenever he consumes any food or drink. The sweat pours down his face and neck, soaking his shirt and requiring a towel to mop up the moisture. He also suffers from hypertension and angina. Latest results include fasting BG 6.9 mmol/l, HbA1c 7.5%, creatinine 224 µmol/l, BP 128/76 mmHg on ramipril 10 mg daily, atenolol 50 mg daily, bendroflumethiazide (bendrofluazide) 2.5 mg daily and simvastatin 20 mg daily. What is the cause of his problem?

### Comment

He is suffering from gustatory sweating, which is a rare form of autonomic neuropathy – most patients also have evidence of other complications. It is difficult to treat. Propantheline bromide is recommended but is rarely tolerated because of side effects. Topical glycopyrrolate cream has been reported to improve symptoms. In some cases symptoms resolve following renal transplant.

Gustatory sweating is a recognised complication of surgical section of the auriculo-temporal nerve when aberrant regrowth results in innervation of the sweat glands in the face by fibres from the vagus nerve. A similar process is thought to occur when diabetes has damaged the nerve function. The patient needs a clear explanation and sympathy, as it is a difficult problem to live with.

### 16.12 What is the prognosis for autonomic neuropathy?

The condition is variable in its natural history and does not inevitably deteriorate. Several studies have found that individual symptoms may remain static over many years, but a few patients clearly deteriorate and some others improve. Often symptomatic episodes, such as diarrhoea or severe postural hypotension, are intermittent and resolve spontaneously.

Patients with autonomic neuropathy have a poor long-term prognosis and in some series below 50% 5-year survival, though it now appears that much of this relates to other complications such as co-existent nephropathy. These patients are at risk in the peri-operative period as they respond poorly to hypoxia and may have cardiac rhythm problems – ECG monitoring is mandatory.

## PRESSURE EFFECTS

### 16.13 What about 'pressure palsies' in diabetes?

Lesions such as carpal tunnel syndrome (*Case vignette 16.3*) appear to be commoner in diabetes, especially type 1, though there are few good controlled data. It is wise to advise patients to avoid pressure on potential pressure points (e.g. elbows, crossed legs, etc.).

### CASE VIGNETTE 16.3

An obese 45-year-old woman with type 1 diabetes for 23 years complains of painful tingling in her fingers. Her latest HbA1c is 7.2% on a three-times daily insulin regimen of Humulin N and Humalog. Detailed questioning suggests it is much worse at night. What is the cause of her symptoms and how can this be managed?

*Comment*

Diabetic neuropathy is unlikely to be the cause of her symptoms if there is no involvement of the legs. If a history and physical examination found no such evidence, then an alternative diagnosis is almost certain. The commonest reason for this patient's symptoms is carpal tunnel syndrome due to pressure on the median nerve at the wrist, which is commoner in diabetes, especially type 1.

Peripheral neuropathy in the hands due to diabetes is usually only seen in very severe cases, where the commonest sign is wasting of the small muscles; for some reason this appears to be commoner with patients with severe nephropathy.

# Diabetic foot and peripheral arterial disease

# 17

The questions here overlap with topics in Chapter 16 (Neuropathy) and also with topics in Chapter 13 (Macrovascular disease).

## DEFINITION AND EPIDEMIOLOGY

### 17.1 What is diabetic foot disease?

It is a complex disease process where varying degrees of peripheral neuropathy and peripheral arterial disease (PAD) cause ischaemia and infection, often aggravated by trauma and physical factors that lead to ulceration and damage to the foot. The end result causes substantial patient morbidity, and amputation may be the final outcome.

In most instances two or more of these factors are present, and may be magnified by poor self-management and/or delay in active intervention.[1-3]

### 17.2 How common are foot lesions and how often do they occur?

Foot disease can be divided into predominantly neuropathic cases or those with neuropathy plus ischaemia – these groups are usually seen in roughly equal proportions. There are also occasional individuals with purely ischaemic lesions. The prevalence figures in *Question 17.3* do not distinguish between type 1 and type 2 patients, and are probably an overestimate for type 2 diabetes.

According to several studies, significant sensory peripheral neuropathy (which leads to loss of normal sensation in the foot) is reported to occur in 10–40% of people with diabetes – lower prevalence rates occur in community-based studies.[4,5] As well as the potential for unperceived injury, neuropathy can also result in abnormal mechanical loading of the feet and subsequent foot deformity, at its most severe in the 'Charcot foot' (*see Q. 17.11*).

### 17.3 How common is peripheral vascular disease in diabetes?

The prevalence of peripheral arterial disease (PAD, a better term than vascular disease) is at least 10–20%, though again exact definitions, tests and populations vary substantially. PAD is several times more common in type 2 diabetes than in non-diabetic populations, and the pattern of arterial disease is frequently more diffuse than in non-diabetic groups – arterial calcification is also commonly seen on X-ray. It often extends to smaller arteries below the knee, though this is not really 'small vessel disease' in the sense of the 'microcirculation'. Ischaemia is caused by reduced blood flow from the arterial disease, and may be compounded by superficial shunting from the arterial to the venous circulation, a common feature of peripheral neuropathy.

## CAUSES AND RISK FACTORS

### 17.4 What are the common causes of foot lesions?

Trauma of various sorts (e.g. stepping on sharp objects, abrasions from poorly fitting shoes, unperceived burns or cracked skin from rubbing callus) is a frequent factor in the breakdown of integrity of the skin or ulcer (*Fig. 17.1*); this provides a portal for the entry of infection. Rapid spread of infection is particularly common in those with diabetes. It is often secondary infection rather than pure ischaemia that leads to gangrene. The infective inflammatory process leads to thrombosis in narrowed small arteries and local areas of gangrene can appear suddenly where circulation was not thought previously to be critical.

Lack of pain, due to neuropathy, frequently contributes to substantial delays in presentation and effective treatment. Foot deformities increase the risk of damage as they alter the normal architecture and pressure-transmitting characteristics, thus enhancing the risk of damage from poorly fitting footwear. Other causes include tinea infections opening up a break in the skin, patient self-treatment and unskilled podiatry.

The main distinguishing characteristics between the different lesions are outlined in *Table 17.1*.

Overall around 5–7% of patients have had a foot ulcer at some stage of their diabetes, more often among older patients and those with long-standing disease.

**TABLE 17.1 Characteristics of foot lesions**

| Neuropathic feet | Neuro-ischaemic feet |
|---|---|
| Warm | Cool |
| Well perfused | Signs of ischaemia |
| Pulses present | Pulses absent or reduced |
| Callus formation | No callus |
| Ulcers usually on soles/pressure points | Ulcers at periphery of feet |
| Usually painless unless active lesion | Possible intermittent claudication or rest pain |

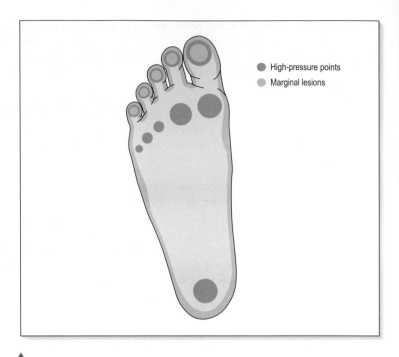

▲

**Fig. 17.1** Diagram of common sites of ulceration. Predominantly neuropathic ulcers occur mainly at points of high pressure (e.g. under metacarpal heads), while ischaemic lesions tend to occur peripherally/marginally. In each case, local deformities, poor-fitting shoes and callus may be major precipitants.

## 17.5 What are the main risk factors for diabetic foot disease?

These include those specifically related to the lower limb, and more general risk factors:

- *Local factors* include the presence of significant peripheral neuropathy and/or significant peripheral arterial disease, the presence of structural foot deformity, plantar callus and/or poor footwear.
- *General factors* include old age, male gender, long duration of diabetes, poor nutritional status/social deprivation, renal disease, reduced mobility/isolation, poor vision and smoking.
- Patients who are at the highest risk of ulceration and amputation include those who have a previous history of foot ulceration or amputation, and peripheral arterial disease.

■ *Previous ulceration* incurs a permanent high risk of future ulceration or amputation so these patients require intensive monitoring. A number of interventions, including follow-up in a specific diabetic foot clinic, specialised footwear and callus debridement, have been shown to reduce ulceration rate.

■ *Previous amputation* is an extremely powerful risk factor for both further ulceration and future amputation. It is also a marker for high mortality; in some series over 60% of patients died within 5 years of the amputation, mainly from cardiovascular disease rather than PAD.

### 17.6 How should these patients be assessed?

There are no reliable symptoms or signs until a late stage in the disease process. Several protocols have been designed to categorise patients as low, moderate or high risk. Screening should be by a trained health professional and the risk assessed on an annual basis.[6,7] Further management can then be based on this assessment, an example of which is the Tayside Assessment Protocol (*Fig. 17.2*).

This assessment should include:

■ *Inspection of the foot*: Inspect the foot for deformity, callus, skin abrasions or local infection (e.g. tinea pedis), standard of self-care, fitting of shoes, current ulceration.

■ *Peripheral neuropathy assessment*: Using 10G monofilaments, neuropathy disability scores or vibration perception threshold are all valuable (*see Q. 16.7*).

■ *Assessment of peripheral circulation*: The presence or absence of dorsalis pedis and posterior tibial pulses assessed by palpation. Absence of pedal pulses, if possible confirmed with Doppler measurements, is a good first-line screen. Symptomatic claudication and/or rest pain are rarely first diagnosed at routine screening (*see Fig. 17.3*).

■ *Ankle/brachial blood pressure ratios*: These may be used, but can be misleading due to arterial calcification – more detailed assessment is best handled by specialists (*see Fig. 17.3*).

■ *Footwear should be checked*. People with established foot disease should be advised to wear high-quality cushioned-sole trainers, those with callus and previous ulceration should have appropriate orthotic footwear.

Once assessed, the recommended supervision is as detailed in *Figure 17.2*.

Patients with diabetes should be assessed annually by a diabetologist, GP, chiropodist, diabetes nurse specialist, or practice nurse with training in diabetes to look for presence of neuropathy, ischaemia or deformity

Patients should be categorised according to the presence of the following symptoms/signs

| Normal sensation AND good pulses AND no previous ulcer AND no foot deformity AND normal vision | Loss of sensation OR absent pulses (or previous vascular surgery) OR significant visual impairment OR physical disability (e.g. stroke, gross obesity) | Previous ulcer due to neuropathy/ischaemia OR Absent pulses and neuropathy OR Callus with risk factor (neuropathy, absent pulse, foot deformity) OR Previous amputation | Active foot ulceration, painful neuropathy which is difficult to control |
|---|---|---|---|
| **LOW RISK** | **MODERATE RISK** | **HIGH RISK** | **ACTIVE FOOT DISEASE** |
| ▽ | ▽ | ▽ | ▽ |
| • No specific regular chiropody input needed (except in exceptional circumstances) • Patients can undertake their own nail care after appropriate education • Annual foot check | Regular (4–12 weekly) general chiropody input advised. For patients with visual impairment or physical disability, who would otherwise fit into the low risk category, input from trained Foot Care Assistants can be substituted (where available) | • Chiropodist with interest and expertise in diabetes either at diabetes unit or in community centre • Chiropodist may want to consider orthotic referral | Suggest making contact with local specialist diabetes team (hospital based) |

In addition, patients with any of the following signs of **ischaemia** or **infection** should be considered for emergency referral to the hospital surgical receiving service or diabetic foot clinic, where appropriate:

| CRITICAL ISCHAEMIA | SEVERE INFECTION |
|---|---|
| • rest or night pain • pale/mottled feet • dependent rubor • ischaemic ulceration • gangrene | • abscess • cellulitis |

**Fig. 17.2** Example protocol for the assessment of risk of the diabetic foot. (Adapted from the Tayside foot risk assessment protocol.)

## INVESTIGATION AND TREATMENT

### 17.7 Is investigation and surgery worthwhile in diabetic patients with peripheral arterial disease?

Recent technical advances in both the diagnosis and surgical treatment of PAD allow more patients to benefit, including those with more distal disease, defined as below the knee.[8] Appropriate techniques include detailed non-invasive vascular studies (*Fig. 17.3*), angiography and subsequent angioplasty, stenting or bypass surgery including distal bypass of smaller vessels below the knee. These have been shown to achieve significant improvements in rates of limb salvage and reduced frequency of amputation.

All patients with tissue loss and PAD should be considered for referral with a view to arterial reconstruction. There is no clear evidence as to the stage at which vascular referral or intervention should take place, but many authorities believe that PAD in diabetes has previously been substantially under-investigated and under-treated.

### 17.8 Are there no medical alternatives?

All patients with PAD require aggressive secondary prevention treatment with aspirin and lipid-lowering therapy. It is important to make sure lipid targets are achieved with treatment (*see Ch. 13*).

Exercise training is valuable in patients with claudication and has been shown to increase claudication distance, but there is little evidence of effective drug therapy though naftidrofuryl (Praxilene) is widely used in the USA. Beta-blockers should be avoided if possible as they substantially reduce claudication distance, which remains a useful measure of severity, progression and functional disability.

### 17.9 How should established ulcers be treated?

Despite these lesions being common, there is little good evidence on optimal treatment.[9] There is, however, widespread expert agreement on certain principles:

- They should be managed by an experienced multi-disciplinary team.[10]
- Early referral, assessment and intervention are vital – infection spreads quickly.
- Early debridement of infected and non-viable tissues is essential.
- There is no evidence of the superiority of any particular antibiotic regimen.
- There is no clear evidence of any particular conventional dressing regimen.
- High-quality cushioned-sole trainers are recommended to allow healing and reduce relapse incidence.[11]
- The greater the vascular problem, the slower and less likely healing will occur.

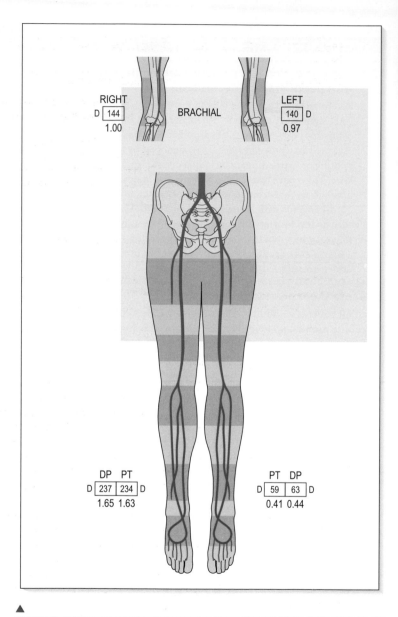

**Fig. 17.3** Detailed non-invasive vascular assessment graphic. The example shows reduction of pressures. The results, from a patient on diet alone, show raised right foot pressure ratios (1.65 and 1.63) suggestive of vascular calcification, but reduced left foot ratios suggestive of significant ischaemia. (Courtesy of Vascular Clinic, Auckland Hospital, Auckland, New Zealand.)

| TABLE 17.2  New interventions in the treatment of established ulcers ||
|---|---|
| Intervention | Evidence and comments |
| Total or similar contact casting | Reduces healing time in appropriate ulcers |
| Growth factors, e.g. becaplermin (Regranex) | Good evidence for speeding or reducing time to healing |
| Living human tissue replacement | Good evidence in selected patients |
| Maggot therapy for debridement | Inconclusive, though some advocates |
| Hyperbaric oxygen | Inconclusive, though some advocates; likely to be more effective if ischaemia is the issue |

■ Associated cellulitis and/or osteomyelitis require immediate hospital assessment/admission.

Several more complex and new therapies have been recommended, though some are expensive, not widely available and/or not fully funded – their use is summarised in *Table 17.2* and in several guidelines.[6]

## COMPLICATIONS

### 17.10 How often does osteomyelitis occur?

Osteomyelitis in the foot is a much-feared complication of diabetic foot ulceration, which results from penetration of infection into bone. It usually results from deep ulcers, though this is often not apparent from superficial examination – careful probing of the wound may be needed. If bone is directly evident on inspection, osteomyelitis should be presumed. Once bone is infected, eradication is extremely difficult, often requiring surgical removal of the affected bone and sometimes amputation. A few cases can be managed by prolonged antibiotic therapy but this needs close specialist supervision.

Proof of the diagnosis is difficult. X-rays only show changes some weeks (perhaps 2–4) after the process has started, though comparison with previous films can be very helpful where available. Patients with foot ulceration should have a foot X-ray at presentation and then at regular intervals if healing is delayed. If deep infection is suspected, the most helpful investigation for both osteomyelitis and deep tissues of the foot is MRI scanning.

### 17.11 What is a 'Charcot foot'?

This is an uncommon complex process where neuropathy and localised osteoporosis lead to fracture and disorganisation of the bones of the foot, which is associated with severe acute inflammation.[12,13] The clinical diagnosis is made, largely by exclusion, based on the following features:

- an erythematous swollen warm foot
- the presence of significant peripheral neuropathy
- the absence of evidence of local infection
- disruption of normal foot architecture, often with loss of the plantar arch.

Pain can be a significant feature in some cases in the early stages. Same-day referral is recommended if the condition is suspected. Investigation may involve thermography, X-ray and, possibly, MRI scanning. Treatment may involve non-weight bearing, total contact casting and the use of bisphosphonates, though the last are not totally proven.

## 17.12 What can be done to prevent ulcers?

There is limited firm evidence but expert opinion suggests the following:
- Footcare education should be part of the multi-disciplinary approach to all people with diabetes.
- Simple foot hygiene – regular inspection, washing and drying; early treatment of any infection (e.g. tinea), abrasion or nail problem.
- All patients with diabetes should be screened annually for foot disease and have a risk assessment.
- Those with high-risk feet or previous ulcers should have access to structured podiatry care.
- Patients with existing disease should be advised to wear high-quality cushioned-sole trainers.

The Tayside protocol (*Fig. 17.2*) gives greater detail of currently recommended care.

**CASE VIGNETTE 17.1**

A man with type 2 diabetes for 10 years, treated with metformin 500 mg twice daily, presents with a new infected dorsal foot ulcer following a blister of his fifth toe caused by an ill-fitting new pair of shoes. The toe looks inflamed and swollen. You are unable to feel any foot pulses in either foot. His latest results from his annual review 1 month ago are as follows: fasting plasma glucose (PG) 9.2 mmol/l, HbA1c 7.7%, total cholesterol 6.1 mmol/l, serum creatinine 69 µmol/l, urine albumin:creatinine ratio 1.9 mg/mmol. An urgent referral to the foot clinic is made and antibiotics are prescribed. What other interventions are required?

*Comment*

This patient's diabetic control is suboptimal and the foot infection is likely to worsen glycaemic control. Close monitoring of diabetes is important and increase in the metformin dosage with possible introduction of a sulphonylurea needs to be considered. When infection is severe and PG levels are markedly disturbed, urgent transfer to insulin therapy will be required. Poor glycaemic control delays healing from infection while continuing infection leads to worsening control! Intensive treatment of both the diabetes and infection is the only way to break the escalating spiral.

This patient also appears to have PAD with absent foot pulses so should be aggressively investigated as healing may be slow without vascular intervention. Additionally he should be treated with aspirin and lipid-lowering therapy.

 **PATIENT QUESTION**

### 17.13  How likely is an amputation?

Though much feared, amputations due to diabetes occur in only a few per cent of patients. They are commoner in those who smoke, those who have multiple complications of their diabetes and those who take least care of themselves.[14]

The best methods of prevention are to avoid smoking, to keep as good as possible control of diabetes and to take regular care of your feet – unlike kidneys and hearts there are as yet no foot transplants!

If there are problems with your feet, see your GP or podiatrist quickly, as delay often leads to rapid worsening of the problem.

# Other complications and accompaniments of diabetes

# 18

## LIVER

### 18.1 Does diabetes cause abnormal liver function tests?

Yes.[1,2] Significant periods of uncontrolled hyperglycaemia, for example as seen at diagnosis of diabetes, can cause markedly raised liver function tests, often two to three times the upper limit of normal. These may reflect the fatty liver associated with hyperglycaemia and the metabolic syndrome and often resolve within weeks or months, assuming reasonable glycaemic control is achieved. Obviously, a full history should be taken including detailed alcohol intake, and other possible causes should be considered – especially if the function tests are more markedly disturbed (> three-fold rises in AST, ALT, GGT, ALP) – or if there is jaundice or signs of clotting or synthetic abnormalities. In the latter situations, diabetes alone is unlikely to be the cause and early investigation/referral including ultrasound is recommended.
Common co-existent or related liver and biliary diseases include:
- Hepatitis A, B or C: B and C are common in Maori and Pacific Island people
- Alcoholic liver disease: probably not commoner
- Haemochromatosis: an uncommon but important secondary cause of diabetes
- Gall stones: commoner in the obese, elderly and possibly diabetes
- Autoimmune liver disease: some types commoner in type 1 diabetes.
Other hepatic disorders may need to be considered with less common ethnic groups and countries of origin, especially in recent immigrants.

### 18.2 Is there usually any underlying clinical liver disease?

'Fatty liver' has been long described in diabetes, and is increasingly being recognised as a common component of the metabolic syndrome.[1,2] Steatohepatitis, the association of an inflammatory infiltrate with fatty liver changes, has recently been recognised and may lead to mild fibrosis and possibly even cirrhosis, though most diabetologists have rarely if ever seen this. It is also known as non-alcoholic fatty liver disease (NAFLD) and non-alcoholic steatohepatitis (NASH). Clinical problems appear to be more common in North America than in the UK, Australia and New Zealand, possibly reflecting the greater degree and frequency of obesity seen in the US – if that is so, we can expect to see more in future years.

Differential diagnosis from alcoholic steatohepatitis is extremely difficult, but beware of labelling a patient with metabolic syndrome as a drinker just on liver function tests! An accurate drinking history is still essential.

Diabetes of any sort can co-exist with any other liver disease without a specific association.

## INFECTIONS

### 18.3 Are infections really commoner in diabetes?

Infections appear commoner in people with diabetes, particularly in the weeks or months before diagnosis and when glycaemic control is poor. Not so clear is whether this is true when glycaemic control is good; the consensus view is that most are not significantly increased in such individuals. There is good laboratory evidence that leucocyte function is impaired with hyperglycaemia above 10–12 mmol/l, which may provide an explanation.

Population studies have confirmed the overall excess of many *bacterial* infections but do not show a higher rate of most *viral* infections such as HIV or sexually transmitted disease; there are, however, a few unusual infections that do appear much commoner (*Table 18.1*).[3,4]

### 18.4 Are dental problems commoner in diabetes?

This is not clear. There is extensive dental (but little medical) literature suggesting this, but selection bias and obesity, diet and socio-economic status have not been controlled for. The problems include xerostomia (dry mouth), initial caries, advanced periodontitis and prosthetic need.

Studies are also conflicting as to whether those with poor glycaemic control, which would presumably encourage dental problems, account for the excess.

**TABLE 18.1 Incidence of infection in diabetes**

| Infections commoner in diabetes* | Rare infections much commoner in diabetes |
|---|---|
| Pyelonephritis/perinephric abscesses | Malignant otitis externa |
| Cellulitis | Rhinocerebral mucomycosis |
| Osteomyelitis/infectious arthritis | Emphysematous infections |
| Rectal and similar abscess formation | |
| Foot infections, especially in deep spaces | |
| Candidiasis | |
| Tuberculosis | |
| Miscellaneous skin infections | |

* Mainly around twice as common.

### 18.5 What about skin infections?

Boils and abscesses are still an occasional presentation of type 2 diabetes, though this is less common now. The same applies to balanitis and vulvitis from Candida infections. In all these instances, it is very difficult to eradicate the infection without obtaining good glycaemic control of the diabetes.

## SKIN AND JOINTS

### 18.6 Are there other specific skin lesions in diabetes?

Yes. Some are virtually specific to diabetes while others are seen with increased frequency or by association:

■ *Acanthosis nigricans* is dark, coarse, thickened skin predominantly seen in flexures and on the neck. Its true association is with insulin resistance and the 'metabolic syndrome' rather than type 2 diabetes per se.
■ *Diabetic dermopathy* is red–brown flat-topped papules.
■ *Necrobiosis lipoidica*, associated with type 1 diabetes, is usually seen over the anterior shin where erythema gives way to a yellowish waxy and atrophic central area which may ulcerate.
■ *Granuloma annulare*, associated mainly with type 1 diabetes, is probably autoimmune in nature and forms partial rings of papules, often on the dorsal surface of hands and feet. It is not exclusive to diabetes.
■ *Xanthelasma and eruptive xanthomata* are not specific to diabetes but are commonly (xanthelasma) or less often (xanthomata) seen in association with lipid derangements. While the former are less specific, often seen around the eyes, eruptive xanthomata are multiple, small, often itchy yellow–white papules often around the buttocks and elbows and usually reflect a severe dyslipidaemia which can also occasionally be seen in the eye as 'lipaemia retinalis'.
■ *Insulin injection site hypertrophy* is a common complication in insulin-treated patients, usually appearing as a soft lump, often with irregular contours. It is due to repetitive injection, often with poor technique, into very localized areas usually because of habit and the lack of discomfort. Repeated use leads to unpredictable insulin absorption with blood glucose (BG) readings fluctuating wildly. It was more commonly seen before the introduction of highly purified insulin but is still a problem in a significant number of people. In any patient using insulin, injection sites should be inspected regularly.

### 18.7 Can joints be affected in diabetes?

There are several conditions that affect joints indirectly, though only gout is a true 'arthritis':

■ *Cheiroarthropathy*, seen in juvenile type 1 diabetes, is actually thickening of collagen around the joints due to glycosylation, and leads to inability to make the 'prayer' sign with the usual complete apposition of hands, joints and fingers. It is usually painless and many patients are unaware of the condition.

■ *Trigger finger and Dupuytren's contracture* are said to be commoner in diabetes; again a possible mechanism is damage to collagen.

■ *Frozen shoulder* is also reputed to be commoner, though evidence is poor.

■ *Gout* is commoner in type 2 diabetes, probably as a major but overlooked component of the metabolic syndrome, particularly common in Maori and Pacific Island patients.

Given the increasing obesity of people with type 2 diabetes, it would not be surprising to see more weight-related disease of the knee, ankle and foot in the future.

## OTHER ORGANS AND IMMUNOLOGICALLY RELATED DISORDERS

### 18.8 What about other organ systems?

Many other systems can be involved, some as a secondary consequence of microvascular disease and some (e.g. as in the lung) have only just been recognised:

■ *Brain*: Limited evidence showing long-term intellectual impairment, possibly vascular in origin.

■ *Lung*: New evidence showing some long-term reduction in lung function.

■ *Gastrointestinal tract*: Coeliac disease and pernicious anaemia commoner in type 1 diabetes; gastroparesis a consequence of autonomic neuropathy; pancreatic cancer commoner (*see Q. 18.11*); diarrhoea, especially nocturnal, a consequence of autonomic neuropathy.

■ *Renal*: Nocturia and frequency, a consequence of hyperglycaemia, often blamed on diabetes, even when well controlled.

■ *Nerve*: Overflow incontinence or urinary retention as consequence of autonomic neuropathy.

■ *Blood*: Clotting factor derangements and platelet abnormalities favouring increased clotting.

### 18.9 Is there more autoimmune disease in diabetes?

It is type 1 diabetes rather than type 2 that shows these associations, with the antigens shown in approximately decreasing order of frequency (*Table 18.2*).

It is less clear whether connective tissue and rheumatological disorders

**TABLE 18.2 Other autoimmune disease in type 1 diabetes**

| Organ | Disease | Antigen | Precise antibody |
|---|---|---|---|
| Thyroid | Primary hypothyroidism | Thyroid peroxidase enzyme | Microsomal antibodies |
| Pancreas | Type 1 diabetes | Islet-cell | Islet cell AB, glutamic acid dehydrogenase |
| Stomach | Pernicious anaemia | Parietal cell, intrinsic factor | ? |
| Ovary | Primary ovarian failure | ? | ? |
| Adrenal cortex | Addison's disease | 21-hydroxylase enzyme | Adrenal cortex |

such as systemic lupus erythematosus and rheumatoid are significantly more common in type 1 or type 2 diabetes. Previous studies may have been flawed because of the inclusion of older type 1 patients (e.g. those with latent autoimmune diabetes in adults) as type 2.

Coeliac disease has recently been found to be associated with type 1, but not type 2, diabetes. The anti-gliadin antibodies may be found in 5% of patients but are not always associated with clinical disease – this should be remembered as a possible cause of weight loss, other gastrointestinal symptoms and anaemia.[5]

## POLYCYSTIC OVARY SYNDROME

### 18.10 Is diabetes related to polycystic ovary syndrome?

Yes, but not in a simple way. Polycystic ovary syndrome (PCOS) is a set of symptoms, not a single disease, and covers several phenotypes.[6] The link appears to be with insulin resistance which is present in many, but not all, patients with PCOS, most of whom are overweight or obese. This is an extremely complex area and the major messages can be summarised as:

■ Some degree of glucose intolerance is very common in these patients.
■ Dyslipidaemia and hypertension are also common, as are other features of the metabolic syndrome.
■ They appear to carry a high risk of macrovascular disease.

In practice, all women with PCOS should be screened for glucose intolerance, metabolic syndrome and cardiovascular risk while young women with diabetes may need evaluation for PCOS if there are any relevant symptoms or complaints (e.g. infertility, oligomenorrhoea or hirsutism).

## CANCER AND OBESITY

### 18.11 Is cancer commoner in diabetes?

Not directly. In nearly all reported mortality studies, deaths from cancer appear to be the same or less than in the general population, with the exception of carcinoma of the pancreas. This may be misleading since chronic pancreatitis may lead to diabetes due to beta-cell insufficiency but is also known to be associated with an increased risk of malignancy. In addition, pancreatic cancer may cause diabetes in its late stages, though it is rarely the presenting feature. Any change in cancer mortality may be because premature deaths from cardiovascular disease have been so much increased in type 2 diabetes, thus 'squeezing out' deaths from cancer which peak at an even older age – this may change in the future (*see also Q. 18.12*).

### 18.12 What are the other associations of obesity itself?

These are many, and potentially increasingly important as weight increases in nearly all populations. Several have clear connections with the metabolic syndrome, and it remains unclear whether they should be considered as core components of that – for example, gout, cholelithiasis, osteoarthrosis, sleep apnoea and polycystic ovary syndrome.

More worrying is a recent report showing an association between obesity and mortality from many cancers in the general population:[7] *Table 18.3* shows which were increased in the most-obese group compared with lean individuals of BMI 18–25 kg/m². It was concluded that 14–20% of US cancer deaths might be attributable to overweight and obesity – as there is normally a long lag period in cancer between the causative agent, presentation and eventual mortality, these figures may continue to grow.

**TABLE 18.3  Increased association between obesity and cancer mortality**

| Men | | Women | |
|---|---|---|---|
| Organ | Increased association | Organ | Increased association |
| Liver | 4.5 fold | Uterus | 6.3 fold |
| Pancreas | 2.6 fold | Kidney | 4.8 fold |
| Stomach | 1.9 fold | Cervix | 3.2 fold |
| Oesophagus | 1.9 fold | Pancreas | 2.8 fold |
| Colon/rectum | 1.8 fold | Oesophagus | 2.6 fold |

# APPENDIX 1
# Stages of change

| Stage | Characteristics of the stage, and suggested interventions |
| --- | --- |
| Pre-contemplation | Denial of a problem (such as the diagnosis of diabetes) or responsibility for a problem. Person not intending to change a specific lifestyle behaviour (diet, physical activity, smoking) in the foreseeable future. A person in this stage may: be reluctant (lack of knowledge), be rebellious (resistant to being told what to do), be resigned (lack energy to make a change), have rationalised (rationalised their existing behaviour to be comfortable with it). *Interventions at this stage:* Develop rapport. Allow the person to express emotions about their diabetes – emotional adjustment to the disease can take many months, and may interfere with the person's ability to process relevant information. Be non-judgemental and non-confrontational. Provide personalised information that is relevant to that individual. Gradually increase the person's perception of the risks from their diabetes, and of the benefits of changing behaviour. |
| Contemplation | Person ambivalent about changing behaviour. A person in this stage is thinking about change but has not yet set a plan of action. 'I would like to get more exercise ... but ...' *Interventions at this stage:* Encourage support networks. Give positive feedback about the person's ability to change. Talk about the pros and cons of the current behaviour and the pros and cons of change. Emphasise the expected benefits of change versus the risks of not changing (tip the balance in favour of change). |
| Preparation | A plan of action is being made and some behaviour change may have taken place. Person is actively getting ready to change the behaviour, and may have taken small steps to change, for example looking for information on walking shoes, healthy nutrition or stress management. |

|  | *Interventions at this stage*:<br>Encourage the person to set specific, achievable goals (e.g. to walk briskly for 30 minutes at least three times a week). Positively reinforce small changes that the person may already have achieved. |
|---|---|
| Action | Busy making changes.<br>*Interventions at this stage*:<br>Refer to an education programme for self-management skills (e.g. a diabetes education programme). Provide self-help materials. |
| Maintenance | Consistent change in pattern of behaviour for at least 6 months. The new behaviour has become a normal way of life and is ingrained in the person's lifestyle. However, relapse is still possible.<br>*Interventions at this stage*:<br>Encourage the person to anticipate and plan ahead for potential difficulties (e.g. maintaining dietary changes while on holiday). Collect information about local resources, such as support groups and supermarket tours. |
| Relapse | Relapse is a temporary stop to the behaviour change process. The length of the stop depends on anticipating the likelihood of relapse and the development of relapse strategies. It is important to avoid a complete stop in the behaviour change process.<br>*Interventions at this stage*:<br>Normalise it – it is very common and understandable. Be non-judgemental about a relapse. Encourage the person to re-enter the stages of change without becoming stuck or demoralised. |

Adapted from Snoek FJ, Skinner TC. Psychological counselling in problematic diabetes: does it help? Diabetic Medicine 2002; 19(4): 265–273.

# APPENDIX 2
# Smoking cessation

## The Five A's:  Ask, Assess, Advise, Assist, Arrange

### I. Ask
The smoking status of every adult should be identified and prominently documented in the medical record. For current smokers and those who have quit in the past year, smoking status should be updated at each visit.

### II. Assess
Determine the willingness of smokers to make a quit attempt, by asking every smoker questions to determine readiness to make a quit attempt.

### III. Advise
Provide brief cessation messages at nearly every encounter. These messages should be:

- clear, strong and personalized
- supportive
- non-confrontational.

### IV. Assist
Provide assistance according to the person's readiness to quit. Relevant information is important for everyone, even those not ready to quit. Provide additional support for those with some interest in quitting:

- Offer self-help material.
- Assist in setting a quit date.
- Help to develop a quit plan.
- Provide practical counselling and support.
- Explore barriers to successful cessation and strategise solutions.
- Offer referral to organised cessation support (e.g. in the UK, the free QUITLINE – 0800 778 778).
- Encourage nicotine replacement therapy (NRT) as first line pharmacotherapy; for previous failure or contraindication to NRT, discuss use of buproprion.

*V. Arrange (follow-up)*

Arrange appropriate follow-up for all smokers. Arrange follow-up (in person or by phone) with smokers who are ready to quit:

■ First follow-up within the first week
■ Second follow-up within the first month
■ Reinforce staying quit during visits in the first year post cessation.

(From *Guidelines on Smoking Cessation, May 2002*, with permission from the National Health Committee, Wellington, New Zealand.)

# APPENDIX 3
## Useful resources

All the websites referred to here were accessed and the addresses checked in April 2004. As internal site organisation changes frequently, we have generally used the home page address as this is likely to remain constant.

If any don't work, first check your spelling and typing! If they still don't, then search on Google etc. using the exact names given plus the relevant country suffix, for example '.uk'.

There are increasing numbers of diabetes-related websites available for many different purposes, though of varying quality. Most of the patients and professional organisations have excellent and extensive link pages to multiple different resources, though we obviously cannot guarantee or endorse the contents of any website!

The following is only a small example of what is available.

### PATIENT AND PROFESSIONAL ORGANISATIONS

*United Kingdom*

**Diabetes UK** (*Patient and Professional*)
10 Parkway
London NW1 7AA
Tel: (+44) (0)20 7424 1819
Fax: (+44) (0)20 7424 1001
E-mail: info@diabetes.org.uk
www.diabetes.org.uk

**MedicAlert** (*Patient*)
1 Bridge Wharf
156 Caledonian Road
London N1 9UU
Freephone 0800 581420
www.medicalert.org

*International organisation with bases in many countries. Sells bracelets and necklaces which alert about medical conditions.*

*Australia*
**Diabetes Australia** (*Patient*)
Level 5, Open Systems House
39 London Circuit
Canberra City ACT 2600

Tel: (+61) (0)2 6232 3800
E-mail: admin@diabetesaustralia.com.au
www.diabetesaustralia.com.au

**Australian Diabetes Society (ADS)** (*Professional*)
145 Macquarie Street
Sydney NSW 2000
Tel: (+61) (0)2 9256 5462
Fax: (+61) (0)2 9251 8174
www.racp.edu.au/ads

*New Zealand*
**Diabetes New Zealand** (*Patient*)
115 Molesworth Street
PO Box 12 441
Wellington 6001
Tel: (+64) (0)4 499 7145
Fax: (+64) (0)4 499 7146
E-mail: diabetes@diabetes.org.nz
www.diabetes.org.nz

**New Zealand Society for the Study of Diabetes (NZSSD)** (*Professional*)
c/o Auckland Diabetes Centre
Greenlane Clinical Centre
Greenlane, Auckland 1005
Tel: (+64) (0)4 499 7145
Fax: (+64) (0)4 499 7146
E-mail: nzssd@diabetes.org.nz
www.diabetes.org.nz

*Europe*
**European Association for the Study of Diabetes (EASD)** (*Professional*)
Rheindorfer Weg 3
D-40591 Düsseldorf
Germany
Tel: (+49) 211 758 4690
Fax: (+49) 211 7584 6929
E-mail: secretariat@easd.org
www.easd.org

*Canada*
**Canadian Diabetes Association (CDA)** (*Patient and Professional*)
15 Toronto Street, Suite 800
Toronto, Ontario M5C 2E3

Tel: (+1) 416 363 0177
Fax: (+1) 416 363 8335
E-mail: info@diabetes.ca
www.diabetes.ca

*United States of America*
**American Diabetes Association** (*Patient*)
1701 North Beauregard Street
Alexandria, VA 22311
Tel: (+1) 703 549 1500
Fax: (+1) 703 549 1715
E-mail: webmaster@diabetes.org
www.diabetes.org

*South Africa*
**South African Diabetes Association** (*Patient*)
PO Box 604
2032 Fontaine Bleau
Tel: (+27) (0) 11 788 4595
E-mail: national@diabetessa.za
www.diabetes.co.za

**INTERNATIONAL ORGANISATIONS**
**International Diabetes Federation (IDF)**
Avenue Emile De Mot 19
1000 Brussels, Belgium
Tel: (+32) (0)2 538 5511
Fax: (+32) (0)2 538 5114
E-mail: info@idf.org
www.idf.org

**World Health Organization (WHO)**
Multiple addresses, details via website: www.who.int

**NATIONAL AND INTERNATIONAL GUIDELINES**
■ Guidelines for guidelines (for diabetes) – downloadable as .pdf files from www.idf.org.
■ Some material from both WHO and IDF as above.

*UK national*
■ SIGN (Wide-ranging full process) – www.sign.ac.uk
■ RCGP (Limited range) – www.rcgp.org.uk
■ NICE (Increasing range, though many inherited) – www.nice.org.uk

*Other national guidelines/recommendations*
- NZGG (Recent [late 2003] wide-ranging derived guideline) – www.nzgg.org.nz
- CDA (Recent [late 2003] online full process) – www.diabetes.ca
- Australian (Extensive range of full-process material) – www.diabetes.net.au
- American (Practice recommendations, not guidelines) – www.diabetes.org

## DIABETES JOURNALS

Many of the major diabetes clinical papers are published in the *New England Journal of Medicine, Lancet or BMJ* and similar general medical journals. The main specialist clinical journals for diabetes (some of which are available online) are:

- *Diabetic Medicine* – Clinical diabetes with a UK/European slant; includes an excellent Continuing Education supplement about 3–4 times annually (www.blackwellscience.com/dme)
- *Diabetes Care* – Clinical diabetes with an American slant (www.diabetesjournals.org)
- *Diabetes et Metabolism*
- *Diabetes Research and Clinical Practice*
- *Practical Diabetes International*

  The main diabetes general practice and education journals are:

- *Diabetes and Primary Care* – UK-based journal matching its title (www.dspace.dial.pipex.com/sbcomm)
- *Journal of Diabetes Nursing* – UK based and practical
- *Diabetes Educator* – American based, strong on educational theory etc. The main scientific journals, in addition to *Nature, Cell* and *JCI* are
- *Diabetes* – American based (www.diabetesjournals.org)
- *Diabetologia* – European

## MAJOR DIABETES PHARMACEUTICAL COMPANIES

Local addresses and contact details are available in national formularies e.g. *BNF*, and virtually all have websites which include local content and contact details. All are in 'www.companyname.com' format, e.g. www.novo-nordisk.com.

- Aventis
- Eli Lilly
- GlaxoSmithKline (GSK)
- Novo Nordisk
- Pfizer (includes Pharmacia)
- Servier

## PATIENT AND PROFESSIONAL WEBSITES

*Patient websites*

Most importantly, the relevant national association websites as listed above are then linked to pages within those sites. There are many others, of which the following deserve mention:

- Diabetes Monitor – www.diabetesmonitor.com
- Diabetes Insight – www.diabetes-insight.info
- Patient UK – www.patient.co.uk/showdoc.asp?doc=246

*Professional websites*

### Literature searching

- Pubmed – www.ncbi.nlm.nih.gov/PubMed
- Medscape – www.medscape.com
- National Electronic Library for Health – www.nelh.nhs.uk

### Academic review sites and similar

- Cochrane – www.update-software.com/cochrane
- Diabetes for Professionals (Novo Nordisk) – www.d4pro.com
- National Institute for Diabetes, Digestive and. Kidney Diseases (US) – www.diabetes.niddk.nih.gov
- Tripdatabase – www.update-software.com
- UKPDS website – www.dtu.ox.ac/ukpds
- Up-to-Date (Subscription medical site) – www.uptodate.com
- Warwick Diabetes Care – www2.warwick.ac.uk/fac/med/diabetes

## Chapter 1

1. Diabetes Prevention Program Research Group. Reduction in the incidence of type 2 diabetes with lifestyle intervention or metformin. New England Journal of Medicine 2002; 346: 393–403.

2. Colman PG, Thomas DW, Zimmet PZ, et al. New classification and criteria for diagnosis of diabetes mellitus. Position statement. Australian Diabetes Society, New Zealand Society for the Study of Diabetes, Royal College of Pathologists of Australasia and Australasian Association of Clinical Biochemists. New Zealand Medical Journal 1999; 112: 139–141.

3. Alberti KG, Zimmet PZ. Definition, diagnosis and classification of diabetes mellitus and its complications. Part 1. Diagnosis and classification of diabetes mellitus: provisional report of a WHO consultation. Diabetic Medicine 1998; 15(7): 539–553.

4. Expert Committee on the Diagnosis and Classification of Diabetes Mellitus. Report of the Expert Committee on the Diagnosis and Classification of Diabetes Mellitus. Diabetes Care 1997; 20: 1183–1197.

5. Unwin N, Shaw J, Zimmet P, et al. Impaired glucose tolerance and impaired fasting glycaemia: the current status on definition and intervention. Diabetic Medicine 2002; 19(9): 708–723.

6. Dunstan DW, Zimmet PZ, Welborn TA, et al. The rising prevalence of diabetes and impaired glucose tolerance. The Australian Diabetes, Obesity and Lifestyle Study. Diabetes Care 2002; 25: 829–834.

7. The cost-effectiveness of screening for type 2 diabetes. CDC Diabetes Cost-Effectiveness Study Group, Centers for Disease Control and Prevention. JAMA 1998; 280(20): 1757–1763.

8. Higson N. Screening for diabetes in general practice. Population screening for diabetes is cost effective. BMJ 2002; 324(7334): 426.

9. Wareham NJ, Griffin SJ. Should we screen for type 2 diabetes? Evaluation against National Screening Committee criteria. BMJ 2001; 322(7292): 986–988.

10. Department of Health. National Service Framework for Diabetes: delivery strategy. London: Department of Health; 2002.

11. Balkau B, Charles MA, Drivsholm T, et al. Frequency of the WHO metabolic syndrome in European cohorts, and an alternative definition of an insulin resistance syndrome. Diabetes Metabolism 2002; 28(5): 364–376.

12. Ford ES, Giles WH. A comparison of the prevalence of the metabolic syndrome using two proposed definitions. Diabetes Care 2003; 26(3): 575–581.

13. Ford ES, Giles WH, Dietz WH. Prevalence of the metabolic syndrome among US adults: findings from the third National Health and Nutrition Examination Survey. JAMA 2002; 287(3): 356–359.

14. Haffner SM. Obesity and the metabolic syndrome: the San Antonio Heart Study. British Journal of Nutrition 2000; 83(Suppl 1): S67–70.

15. Davies MJ, Gray IP. Impaired glucose tolerance. BMJ 1996; 312: 264–265.

16. Keen H, Jarrett RJ, McCartney P. The ten-year follow-up of the Bedford survey (1962–1972): glucose tolerance and diabetes. Diabetologia 1982; 22(2): 73–78.

17. Tuomilehto J, Lindstrom J, Eriksson JG, et al. Prevention of type 2 diabetes mellitus by changes in lifestyle among subjects with impaired glucose tolerance. New England Journal of Medicine 2001; 344(18): 1343–1350.

18. Pan X, Li G, Hu Y, et al. Effects of diet and exercise in preventing NIDDM in people with impaired glucose tolerance. The Da Qing IGT and Diabetes Study. Diabetes Care 1997; 20: 537–544.

19. Torgerson JS, Hauptman J, Boldrin MN, Sjostrom L. XENical in the prevention of diabetes in obese subjects (XENDOS) study: a randomized study of orlistat as an adjunct to lifestyle changes for the prevention of type 2 diabetes in obese patients. Diabetes Care 2004; 27(1): 155–161.

20. Chiasson J-L, Josse RG, Gomis R, et al. Acarbose treatment and the risk of cardiovascular disease and hypertension in patients with impaired glucose tolerance: The STOP-NIDDM Trial. JAMA 2003; 290(4): 486–494.

21. Colditz GA, Willett WC, Rotnitzky A, et al. Weight gain as a risk factor for clinical diabetes mellitus in women. Annals of Internal Medicine 1995; 122(7): 481–486.

22. Gatling W, Guzder RN, Turnbull JC, et al. The Poole Diabetes Study: how many cases of Type 2 diabetes are diagnosed each year during normal health care in a defined community? Diabetes Res Clin Pract 2001; 3(2): 107–112.

23. Alberti KG, Gray DP. The care of diabetes. Diabetic Medicine 1998; 15(Suppl 3): S3–4.

24. World Health Organization. Definition, diagnosis and classification of diabetes mellitus and its complications. Geneva: WHO; 1999.

25. Ford ES, Giles WH. A comparison of the prevalence of the metabolic syndrome using two proposed definitions. Diabetes Care 2003; 26(3): 575–581.

26. Laaksonen DE, Lakka HM, Niskanen LK, et al. Metabolic syndrome and development of diabetes mellitus: application and validation of recently suggested definitions of the metabolic syndrome in a prospective cohort study. American Journal of Epidemiology 2002; 156(11): 1070–1077.

27. Devendra D, Liu E, Eisenbarth GS. Type 1 diabetes: recent developments. BMJ 2004; 328(7442): 750–754.

28. Gale EA, Bingley PJ, Emmett CL, et al. European Nicotinamide Diabetes Intervention Trial (ENDIT): a randomised controlled trial of intervention before the onset of type 1 diabetes. Lancet 2004; 363: 925–931.

29. Petersen KF, Dufour S, Belfroy D, et al. Impaired mitochondrial activity in the insulin-resistant offspring of patients with type 2 diabetes. New England Journal of Medicine 2004; 350(7): 664–671.

30. Taylor R. Causation of type 2 diabetes – the Gordian knot unravels. New England Journal of Medicine 2004; 350(7): 639–641.

31. Mogensen CE, Cooper ME. Diabetic renal disease: from recent studies to improved clinical practice. Diabetic Medicine 2004; 21(1): 4–17.

32. Cooper M, Boner G. Dual blockade of the renin-angiotensin system in diabetic nephropathy. Diabetic Medicine 2004; 21(s1): 15–18.

33. Bilous RW. End-stage renal failure and management of diabetes. Diabetic Medicine 2004; 21(s1): 12–14.

## Chapter 2

1. UK Prospective Diabetes Study (UKPDS) Group. Intensive blood-glucose control with sulphonylureas or insulin compared with conventional treatment and risk of complications in patients with type 2 diabetes (UKPDS 33). Lancet 1998; 352: 837–853.

2. The Diabetes Control and Complications Trial Research Group. The effect of intensive treatment of diabetes on the development and progression of long-term complications in insulin-dependent diabetes mellitus. New England Journal of Medicine 1993; 329(14): 977–986.

3. Ohkubo Y, Kishikawa H, Araki E, et al. Intensive insulin therapy prevents the progression of diabetic microvascular complications in Japanese patients with non-insulin-dependent diabetes mellitus: a randomized prospective 6-year study. (Kumamoto Study). Diabetes Research and Clinical Practice 1995; 28: 103–117.

4. UK Prospective Diabetes Study (UKPDS) Group. Effect of intensive blood-glucose control with metformin on complications in overweight patients with type 2 diabetes (UKPDS 34). Lancet 1998; 352: 854–865.

5. UK Prospective Diabetes Study (UKPDS) Group. Tight blood pressure control and risk of macrovascular and microvascular complications in type 2 diabetes (UKPDS 38). BMJ 1998; 317(7160): 703–713.

6. Adler AI, Stratton IM, Neil HA, et al. Association of systolic blood pressure with macrovascular and microvascular complications of type 2 diabetes (UKPDS 36): prospective observational study. BMJ 2000; 321(7258): 412–419.

7. Stratton IM, Adler AI, Neil HAW, et al. Association of glycaemia with macrovascular and microvascular complications of type 2 diabetes (UKPDS 35): prospective observational study. BMJ 2000; 321: 405–412.

8. Wang PH, Lau J, Chalmers TC. Meta-analysis of effects of intensive blood-glucose control on late complications of type 1 diabetes. Lancet 1993; 341(8856): 1306–1309.

9. The QuED Study Group. Attitudes of Italian physicians towards intensive metabolic control in type 2 diabetes. The QuED Study Group – Quality of Care and Outcomes in Type 2 Diabetes. Diabetes Nutrition and Metabolism 2000; 13(3): 149–155.

10. Australian Centre for Diabetes Strategies. National evidence based guidelines for the management of type 2 diabetes. Sydney: Diabetes Australia Guideline Development Consortium; 2000.

11. Scottish Intercollegiate Guidelines Network. Management of diabetes: a national clinical guideline. Edinburgh: Royal College of Physicians; 2001.

12. New Zealand Guidelines Group. Management of type 2 diabetes. Wellington: New Zealand Guidelines Group; 2003.

13. Winocour PH. Effective diabetes care: a need for realistic targets. BMJ 2002; 324(7353): 1577–1580.

14. McAulay V, Deary IJ, Frier BM. Symptoms of hypoglycaemia in people with diabetes. Diabetic Medicine 2001; 18(9): 690–705.

15. de Galan BE, Hoekstra JB. Glucose counterregulation in type 2 diabetes mellitus. Diabetic Medicine 2001; 18(7): 519–527.

16. The Diabetes Control and Complications Trial Research Group. Clustering of long-term complications in families with diabetes in the diabetes control and complications trial. Diabetes 1997; 46(11): 1829–1839.

17. Henricsson M, Nilsson A, Groop L, et al. Prevalence of diabetic retinopathy in relation to age at onset of the diabetes, treatment, duration and glycemic control. Acta Ophthalmologica Scandinavica 1996; 74: 523–527.

18. Klein R, Klein BE, Moss SE, et al. The Wisconsin epidemiologic study of diabetic retinopathy II. Prevalence and risk of diabetic retinopathy when age at diagnosis is less than 30 years. Archives of Ophthalmology 1984; 102: 520–526.

19. Klein R, Klein BE, Moss SE, et al. The Wisconsin epidemiologic study of diabetic retinopathy III. Prevalence and risk of diabetic retinopathy when age at diagnosis is 30 or more years. Archives of Ophthalmology 1984; 102: 527–532.

20. Tapp RJ, Shaw JE, Harper CA, et al. The prevalence of and factors associated with diabetic retinopathy in the Australian population. Diabetes Care 2003; 26(6): 1731–1737.

21. Adler AI, Stevens RJ, Manley SE, et al. Development and progression of nephropathy in type 2 diabetes: the United Kingdom Prospective Diabetes Study (UKPDS 64). Kidney International 2003; 63(1): 225–232.

22. Laing SP, Swerdlow AJ, Slater SD, et al. Mortality from heart disease in a cohort of 23,000 patients with insulin-treated diabetes. Diabetologia 2003; 46(6): 760–765.

## Chapter 4

1. Bonow RO, Eckel RH. Diet, obesity, and cardiovascular risk. New England Journal of Medicine 2003; 348(21): 2057–2058.

2. Mann JI. Diet and risk of coronary heart disease and type 2 diabetes. Lancet 2002; 360(9335): 783–789.

3. Trichopoulou A, Costacou T, Bamia C, et al. Adherence to a Mediterranean diet and survival in a Greek population. New England Journal of Medicine 2003; 348(26): 2599–2608.

4. de Lorgeril M, Salen P, Martin JL, et al. Mediterranean diet, traditional risk factors, and the rate of cardiovascular complications after myocardial infarction: final report of the Lyon Diet Heart Study. Circulation 1999; 99(6): 779–785.

5. Frost G, Dornhorst A. The relevance of the glycaemic index to our understanding of dietary carbohydrates. Diabetic Medicine 2000; 17(5): 336–345.

6. Brand-Miller J, Hayne S, Petocz P, et al. Low-glycemic index diets in the management of diabetes: a meta-analysis of randomized controlled trials. Diabetes Care 2003; 26(8): 2261–2267.

7. DAFNE Study Group. Training in flexible, intensive insulin management to enable dietary freedom in people with type 1 diabetes: dose adjustment for normal eating (DAFNE) randomised controlled trial. BMJ 2002; 325(7367): 746–748.

8. Noel PH, Pugh JA. Management of overweight and obese adults. BMJ 2002; 325(7367): 757–761.

9. Mertens IL, Van Gaal LF. Overweight, obesity, and blood pressure: the effects of modest weight reduction. Obesity Research 2000; 8(3): 270–278.

10. Stewart KJ. Exercise training and the cardiovascular consequences of type 2 diabetes and hypertension: plausible mechanisms for improving cardiovascular health. JAMA 2002; 288(13): 1622–1631.

11. Boule NG, Haddad E, Kenny GP, et al. Effects of exercise on glycemic control and body mass in type 2 diabetes mellitus: a meta-analysis of controlled clinical trials. JAMA 2001; 286(10): 1218–1227.

12. Anonymous. Diabetes mellitus and exercise. Diabetes Care 2001; 24 (Suppl 1): S51–S55.

13. Haire-Joshu D, Glasgow RE, Tibbs TL. Smoking and diabetes. Diabetes Care 1999; 22(11): 1887–1898.

14. Neaton JD, Wentworth D. Serum cholesterol, blood pressure, cigarette smoking, and death from coronary heart disease. Overall findings and differences by age for 316,099 white men. Multiple Risk Factor Intervention Trial Research Group. Archives of Internal Medicine 1992; 152(1): 56–64.

15. National Health Committee. Guidelines for smoking cessation (revised May 2002). Wellington: New Zealand Guidelines Group, National Health Committee; 2002.

16. Taylor MD, Frier BM, Gold AE, et al. Psychosocial factors and diabetes-related outcomes following diagnosis of Type 1 diabetes in adults: the Edinburgh Prospective Diabetes Study. Diabetic Medicine 2003; 20(2): 135–146.

17. Recommendations for the nutritional management of patients with diabetes mellitus. European Journal of Clinical Nutrition 2000; 54(4): 353–355.

## Chapter 5

1. De Fronzo R, Goodman A. Efficacy of metformin in patients with non-insulin-dependent diabetes mellitus. The Multicenter Metformin Study Group. New England Journal of Medicine 1995; 333(9): 541–549.

2. De Fronzo RA. Pharmacologic therapy for type 2 diabetes mellitus. Annals of Internal Medicine 1999; 131(4): 281–303.

3. Krentz AJ, Bailey CJ, Melander A. Thiazolidinediones for type 2 diabetes. New agents reduce insulin resistance but need long term clinical trials. BMJ 2000; 321(7256): 252–253.

4. Day C. Thiazolidinediones: a new class of antidiabetic drugs. Diabetic Medicine 1999; 16(3): 179–192.

5. Wagstaff AJ, Goa KL. Rosiglitazone: a review of its use in the management of type 2 diabetes mellitus. Drugs 2002; 62(12): 1805–1837.

6. Leibowitz GP, Cerasi EP. Sulphonylurea treatment of NIDDM patients with cardiovascular disease: a mixed blessing? Diabetologia 1996; 39(5): 503–514.

7. Hermann LS, Schersten B, Melander A. Antihyperglycaemic efficacy, response prediction and dose–response relations of treatment with metformin and sulphonylurea, alone and in primary combination. Diabetic Medicine 1994; 11: 953–960.

8. Dornhorst A. Insulinotropic meglitinide analogues. Lancet 2001; 358(9294): 1709–1716.

9. Owens DR. Repaglinide – prandial glucose regulator: a new class of oral antidiabetic drugs. Diabetic Medicine 1998; 15(Suppl 4): S28–36.

10. Chiasson J-L, Josse RG, Gomis R, et al. Acarbose treatment and the risk of cardiovascular disease and hypertension in patients with impaired glucose tolerance: the STOP-NIDDM trial. JAMA 2003; 290(4): 486–494.

11. Kelley DE, Bidot P, Freedman Z, et al. Efficacy and safety of acarbose in insulin-treated patients with type 2 diabetes. Diabetes Care 1998; 21: 2056–2061.

12. UK Prospective Diabetes Study (UKPDS) Group. Effect of intensive blood-glucose control with metformin on complications in overweight patients with type 2 diabetes (UKPDS 34). Lancet 1998; 352: 854–865.

13. Bailey C, Turner R. Metformin. New England Journal of Medicine 1996; 334(9): 574–579.

14. Jones GC, Macklin JP, Alexander WD. Contraindications to the use of metformin. BMJ 2003; 326(7379): 4–5.

15. Auwerx JP. PPARgamma, the ultimate thrifty gene. Diabetologia 1999; 42(9): 1033–1049.

16. Gale EA. Lessons from the glitazones: a story of drug development. Lancet 2001; 357(9271): 1870–1875.

17. Van Gaal LF, De Leeuw IH. Rationale and options for combination therapy in the treatment of Type 2 diabetes. Diabetologia 2003; 46(Suppl 1): M44–50.

18. Inzucchi SE. Oral antihyperglycemic therapy for type 2 diabetes: scientific review. JAMA 2002; 287(3): 360–372.

19. Aljabri K, Kozak SE, Thompson DM. Addition of pioglitazone or bedtime insulin to maximal doses of sulfonylurea and metformin in type 2 diabetes patients with poor glucose control: a

prospective, randomized trial. American Journal of Medicine 2004; 116: 230–235.

## Chapter 6

1. Owens DR, Zinman B, Bolli GB. Insulins today and beyond. Lancet 2001; 358(9283): 739–746.

2. Hamann A, Matthaei S, Rosak C, et al. A randomized clinical trial comparing breakfast, dinner, or bedtime administration of insulin glargine in patients with type 1 diabetes. Diabetes Care 2003; 26(6): 1738–1744.

3. Murphy NP, Keane SM, Ong KK, et al. Randomized cross-over trial of insulin glargine plus lispro or NPH insulin plus regular human insulin in adolescents with type 1 diabetes on intensive insulin regimens. Diabetes Care 2003; 26(3): 799–804.

4. McKeage K, Goa K. Insulin glargine: a review of its therapeutic use as a long-acting agent for the management of type 1 and 2 diabetes mellitus. Drugs 2001; 61(11): 1599–1624.

5. Rossetti P, Pampanelli S, Fanelli F, et al. Intensive replacement of basal insulin in patients with type 1 diabetes given rapid-acting analog at mealtime: a 3-month comparison between administration of NPH insulin four times daily or bedtime. Diabetes Care 2003; 26: 1490–1496.

6. Winocour PH. Effective diabetes care: a need for realistic targets. BMJ 2002; 324(7353): 1577–1580.

7. Trewby PN, Reddy AV, Trewby CS, et al. Are preventive drugs preventive enough? A study of patients' expectation of benefits from preventive drugs. Clinical Medicine 2002; 2(6): 527–533.

8. Yki-Jarvinen H, Ryysy L, Nikkila K, et al. Comparison of bedtime insulin regimens in patients with type 2 diabetes mellitus. A randomized, controlled trial. Annals of Internal Medicine 1999; 130(5): 389–396.

9. Puhakainen I, Taskinen M, Yki-Jarvinen H. Comparison of acute daytime and nocturnal insulinization on diurnal glucose homeostasis in NIDDM. Diabetes Care 1994; 17(8): 805–809.

10. Yki-Jarvinen H, Dressler A, Ziemen M. Less nocturnal hypoglycemia and better post-dinner glucose control with bedtime insulin glargine compared with bedtime NPH insulin during insulin combination therapy in type 2 diabetes. HOE 901/3002 Study Group. Diabetes Care 2000; 23(8): 1130–1136.

11. Home PD. Intensive insulin therapy in clinical practice. Diabetologia 1997; 40(Suppl 2): S83–87.

12. Wulffele MG, Kooy A, Lehert P, et al. Combination of insulin and metformin in the treatment of type 2 diabetes. Diabetes Care 2002; 25(12): 2133–2140.

13. Airey CM, Williams DR, Martin PG, et al. Hypoglycaemia induced by exogenous insulin –'human' and animal insulin compared. Diabetic Medicine 2000; 17(6): 416–432.

14. Pickup J, Mattock M, Kerry S. Glycaemic control with continuous subcutaneous insulin infusion compared with intensive insulin injections in patients with type 1 diabetes: meta-analysis of randomised controlled trials. BMJ 2002; 324(7339): 705.

## Chapter 7

1. UK Prospective Diabetes Study (UKPDS) Group. Intensive blood-glucose control with sulphonylureas or insulin compared with conventional treatment and risk of complications in patients with type 2 diabetes (UKPDS 33). Lancet 1998; 352: 837–853.

2. Ohkubo Y, Kishikawa H, Araki E, et al. Intensive insulin therapy prevents the progression of diabetic microvascular complications in Japanese patients with non-insulin-dependent diabetes

mellitus: a randomized prospective 6-year study. (Kumamoto Study). Diabetes Research & Clinical Practice 1995; 28: 103–117.

3. The DCCT Research Group. The effect of intensive treatment of diabetes on the development and progression of long-term complications in insulin-dependent diabetes mellitus. New England Journal of Medicine 1993; 329: 977–986.

4. Dornhorst A. Insulinotropic meglitinide analogues. Lancet 2001; 358(9294): 1709–1716.

5. Cryer PE. Hypoglycaemia: the limiting factor in the glycaemic management of Type I and Type II diabetes. Diabetologia 2002; 45(7): 937–948.

6. Amiel S, Maran A. Hypoglycaemia in insulin-dependent diabetes mellitus: facts for the 1990s. Diabete & Metabolisme 1993; 19(4): 332–339.

7. de Galan BE, Hoekstra JB. Glucose counter-regulation in Type 2 diabetes mellitus. Diabetic Medicine 2001; 18(7): 519–527.

8. Smith D, Amiel SA. Hypoglycaemia unawareness and the brain. Diabetologia 2002; 45(7): 949–958.

9. Cranston I, Lomas J, Maran A, et al. Restoration of hypoglycaemia awareness in patients with long-duration insulin-dependent diabetes. Lancet 1994; 344(8918): 283–287.

10. Amiel S. R.D. Lawrence Lecture 1994. Limits of normality: the mechanisms of hypoglycaemia unawareness. Diabetic Medicine 1994; 11(10): 918–924.

11. Spyer G, Hattersley AT, MacDonald IA, et al. Hypoglycaemic counter-regulation at normal blood glucose concentrations in patients with well controlled type-2 diabetes. Lancet 2000; 356(9246): 1970–1974.

12. MacLeod KM. Diabetes and driving: towards equitable, evidence-based decision-making. Diabetic Medicine 1999; 16(4): 282–290.

13. Herman WH. Clinical evidence: glycaemic control in diabetes. BMJ 1999; 319(7202): 104–106.

## Chapter 8

1. Morris AD, Boyle DI, McMahon AD, et al. Adherence to insulin treatment, glycaemic control, and ketoacidosis in insulin-dependent diabetes mellitus. The DARTS/MEMO Collaboration. Diabetes Audit and Research in Tayside, Scotland. Medicines Monitoring Unit. Lancet 1997; 350(9090): 1505–1510.

2. Ferrannini E, Balkau B. Insulin: in search of a syndrome. Diabetic Medicine 2002; 19(9): 724–729.

3. Surwit RS, van Tilburg MA, Zucker N, et al. Stress management improves long-term glycemic control in type 2 diabetes. Diabetes Care 2002; 25(1): 30–34.

4. Snoek FJ, Skinner TC. Psychological counselling in problematic diabetes: does it help? Diabetic Medicine 2002; 19(4): 265–273.

5. Taylor MD, Frier BM, Gold AE, et al. Psychosocial factors and diabetes-related outcomes following diagnosis of Type 1 diabetes in adults: the Edinburgh Prospective Diabetes Study. Diabetic Medicine 2003; 20(2): 135–146.

6. Trento M, Passera P, Bajardi M, et al. Lifestyle intervention by group care prevents deterioration of type 2 diabetes: a 4-year randomised controlled clinical trial. Diabetologia 2002; 45(9): 1231–1239.

7. Rachmani R, Levi Z, Slavachevski M, et al. Teaching patients to monitor their risk factors retards the progression of vascular complications in high-risk patients with type 2 diabetes mellitus – a randomised prospective study. Diabetic Medicine 2002; 19(5): 385–392.

8. Malmberg K. Prospective randomized study of intensive insulin treatment on long term survival after acute myocardial infarction in patients with diabetes. DIGAMI (Diabetes Mellitus,

Insulin Glucose Infusion in Acute Myocardial Infarction) Study Group. BMJ 1997; 314: 1512–1515.

9. Jones JM, Lawson ML, Daneman D, et al. Eating disorders in adolescent females with and without type 1 diabetes: cross sectional study. BMJ 2000; 320(7249): 1563–1566.

## Chapter 9

1. Metchick LN, Petit WA, Inzucchi SE. Inpatient management of diabetes mellitus. American Journal of Medicine 2002; 113: 317–323.

2. Thomsen HS, Morcos SK. Contrast media and metformin: guidelines to diminish the risk of lactic acidosis in non-insulin-dependent diabetics after administration of contrast media. European Radiology 1999; 9(4): 738–740.

## Chapter 10

1. Department of Health. National Service Framework for Diabetes: Standards. London: Department of Health; 2001.

2. Department of Health. National Service Framework for Diabetes: Delivery strategy. London: Department of Health; 2002.

3. MacKinnon M. Providing diabetes care in general practice: a practical guide for the primary care team, 4th edn. London: Class Publishing; 2002.

4. Levene LS. Management of type 2 diabetes mellitus in primary care: a practical guide. Edinburgh: Butterworth Heinemann; 2003.

5. Morris AD, Boyle DI, MacAlpine R, et al. The diabetes audit and research in Tayside Scotland (DARTS) study: electronic record linkage to create a diabetes register. BMJ 1997; 315(7107): 524–528.

6. Whitford DL, Roberts SH. Electronic record linkage to create diabetes registers. Registers constructed from primary care databases have advantages. BMJ 1998; 316(7129): 472–473.

7. Scottish Intercollegiate Guidelines Network (SIGN). Management of diabetes: a national clinical guideline. SIGN publication no. 55. Edinburgh: SIGN; 2001.

8. Lord J, Paisley S, Taylor R. The clinical effectiveness and cost-effectiveness of rosiglitazone for type 2 diabetes mellitus. London: National Institute for Clinical Excellence; 2000.

9. New Zealand Guidelines Group. Management of type 2 diabetes. Wellington: New Zealand Guidelines Group; 2003.

10. Australian Centre for Diabetes Strategies. National evidence based guidelines for the management of type 2 diabetes. Sydney: Diabetes Australia Guideline Development Consortium; 2000.

11. American Diabetes Association. Clinical practice recommendations 2003. Diabetes Care 2003; 26(Suppl 1): S1–S156.

12. Gaede P, Vedel P, Larsen N, et al. Multifactorial intervention and cardiovascular disease in patients with type 2 diabetes. New England Journal of Medicine 2003; 348(5): 383–393.

13. California Healthcare Foundation/ American Geriatrics Society. Guidelines for improving the care of the older person with diabetes mellitus. Journal of the American Geriatrics Society 2003; 51: S265–280.

14. Australian Diabetes Educators Association. Guidelines for the management and care of diabetes in the elderly. Canberra: ADEA; 2003. (See also www.adea.com.au)

15. Diabetes UK. What diabetes care to expect. London: Diabetes UK; 2003.

## Chapter 11

1. Miles P, Everett J, Murphy J, Kerr D. Comparison of blood or urine testing by

patients with newly diagnosed non-insulin dependent diabetes: patient survey after randomised crossover trial. BMJ 1997; 315: 348–349.

2. Snoek FJ, Skinner TC. Psychological counselling in problematic diabetes: does it help? Diabetic Medicine 2002; 19(4): 265–273.

3. Talbot F, Nouwen A. A review of the relationship between depression and diabetes in adults: is there a link? Diabetes Care 2000; 23: 1556–1562.

4. Lustman PJ, Freedland KE, Griffith LS, et al. Fluoxetine for depression in diabetes: a randomized double-blind placebo-controlled trial. Diabetes Care 2000; 23: 618–623.

5. Surwit RS, van Tilburg MA, Zucker N, et al. Stress management improves long-term glycemic control in type 2 diabetes. Diabetes Care 2002; 25(1): 30–34.

6. From the Centers for Disease Control and Prevention. Influenza and pneumococcal vaccination rates among persons with diabetes mellitus – United States, 1997. JAMA 2000; 283(1): 48–50.

7. MacLeod KM. Diabetes and driving: towards equitable, evidence-based decision-making. Diabetic Medicine 1999; 16(4): 282–290.

8. Edwards R, Burns JA, McElduff P, et al. Variations in process and outcomes of diabetes care by socio-economic status in Salford, UK. Diabetologia 2003; 46(6): 750–759.

9. Yeh G, Eisenberg D, Davis R, et al. Use of complementary and alternative medicine among persons with diabetes mellitus: results of a national survey. American Journal of Public Health 2002; 92(10): 1648–1652.

10. Yeh GY, Eisenberg DM, Kaptchuk TJ, et al. Systematic review of herbs and dietary supplements for glycemic control in diabetes. Diabetes Care 2003; 26(4): 1277–1294.

## Chapter 12

1. Temple R, Aldridge V, Greenwood R, et al. Association between outcome of pregnancy and glycaemic control in early pregnancy in type 1 diabetes: population based study. BMJ 2002; 325(7375): 1275–1276.

2. Casson IF, Clarke CA, Howard CV, et al. Outcomes of pregnancy in insulin dependent diabetic women: results of a five year population cohort study. BMJ 1997; 315(7103): 275–278.

3. Cundy T, Gamble G, Townend K, et al. Perinatal mortality in Type 2 diabetes mellitus. Diabetic Medicine 2000; 17(1): 33–38.

4. Pregnancy outcomes in the Diabetes Control and Complications Trial. American Journal of Obstetrics and Gynecology 1996; 174(4): 1343–1353.

5. Hawthorne G, Irgens LM, Lie RT. Outcome of pregnancy in diabetic women in northeast England and in Norway, 1994–7. BMJ 2000; 321(7263): 730–731.

6. Langer O, Conway D, Berkus M, et al. A comparison of glyburide and insulin in women with gestational diabetes mellitus. New England Journal of Medicine 2000; 343(16): 1134–1138.

7. Vittinghoff E, Shlipak MG, Varosy PD, et al. Risk factors and secondary prevention in women with heart disease: the Heart and Estrogen/Progestin Replacement Study. Annals of Internal Medicine 2003; 138(2): 110.

8. Writing Group for the Women's Health Initiative Investigators. Risks and benefits of estrogen plus progestin in healthy postmenopausal women: principal results from the Women's Health Initiative randomized controlled trial. JAMA 2002; 288: 321–333.

9. Beral V, Banks E, Reeves G. Evidence from randomised trials on the long-term effects of hormone replacement therapy. Lancet 2002; 360(9337): 942–944.

10. Cohan P, Korenman S. Erectile dysfunction. Journal of Clinical Endocrinology and Metabolism 2001; 86(6): 2391–2394.

11. Boulton A, Selam J, Sweeney M, et al. Sildenafil citrate for the treatment of erectile dysfunction in men with Type II diabetes mellitus. Diabetologia 2001; 44(10): 1296–1301.

12. Goldstein I, Young JM, Fischer J, et al. Vardenafil, a new phosphodiesterase type 5 inhibitor, in the treatment of erectile dysfunction in men with diabetes: a multicenter double-blind placebo-controlled fixed-dose study. Diabetes Care 2003; 26(3): 777–783.

## Chapter 13

1. Laing SP, Swerdlow AJ, Slater SD, et al. Mortality from heart disease in a cohort of 23,000 patients with insulin-treated diabetes. Diabetologia 2003; 46(6): 760–765.

2. Solomon CG. Reducing cardiovascular risk in type 2 diabetes. New England Journal of Medicine 2003; 348(5): 457–459.

3. Laakso M. Cardiovascular disease in type 2 diabetes: challenge for treatment and prevention. Journal of Internal Medicine 2001; 249(3): 225–235.

4. Schernthaner G. Cardiovascular mortality and morbidity in type-2 diabetes mellitus. Diabetes Research and Clinical Practice 1996; 31(Suppl): S3–13.

5. Ministry of Health. Modelling diabetes: the mortality burden. Wellington: Ministry of Health; 2002.

6. Carroll C, Naylor E, Marsden P, et al. How do people with Type 2 diabetes perceive and respond to cardiovascular risk? Diabetic Medicine 2003; 20(5): 355–360.

7. Davis TM, Millns H, Stratton IM, et al. Risk factors for stroke in type 2 diabetes mellitus: United Kingdom Prospective Diabetes Study (UKPDS) 29. Archives of Internal Medicine 1999; 159(10): 1097–1103.

8. Gorelick PB, Sacco RL, Smith DB, et al. Prevention of a first stroke: a review of guidelines and a multidisciplinary consensus statement from the National Stroke Association. JAMA 1999; 281(12): 1112–1120.

9. Kuusisto J, Mykkanen L, Pyorala K, et al. Non-insulin-dependent diabetes and its metabolic control are important predictors of stroke in elderly subjects. Stroke 1994; 25(6): 1157–1164.

10. Haffner S, Lehto S, Ronnemaa T. Mortality from coronary disease in subjects with type 2 diabetes and in non-diabetic subjects with and without prior myocardial infarction. New England Journal of Medicine 1998; 339: 229–234.

11. Ridker PM, Rifai N, Rose L, et al. Comparison of C-reactive protein and low-density lipoprotein cholesterol levels in the prediction of first cardiovascular events. New England Journal of Medicine 2002; 347(20): 1557–1565.

12. Prescott SM, Zimmerman GA, McIntyre TM, et al. Inflammation in the vascular wall as an early event in atherosclerosis. Diabetologia 1997; 40(Suppl 2): S111–112.

13. Neaton JD, Wentworth D. Serum cholesterol, blood pressure, cigarette smoking, and death from coronary heart disease. Overall findings and differences by age for 316,099 white men. Multiple Risk Factor Intervention Trial Research Group. Archives of Internal Medicine 1992; 152(1): 56–64.

14. Winocour PH, Fisher M. Prediction of cardiovascular risk in people with diabetes. Diabetic Medicine 2003; 20(7): 515–527.

15. Stratton IM, Adler AI, Neil HAW, et al. Association of glycaemia with macrovascular and microvascular complications of type 2 diabetes (UKPDS 35): prospective observational study. BMJ 2000; 321(7258): 405–412.

16. Game FL, Jones AF. Coronary heart disease risk assessment in diabetes mellitus – a comparison of PROCAM and Framingham risk assessment functions. Diabetic Medicine 2001; 18: 355–359.

17. Cappuccio FP, Oakeshott P, Strazzullo P, et al. Application of Framingham risk estimates to ethnic minorities in United Kingdom and implications for primary prevention of heart disease in general practice: cross sectional population based study. BMJ 2002; 325(7375): 1271.

18. Stevens RJ, Kothari V, Adler AI, et al. The UKPDS risk engine: a model for the risk of coronary heart disease in Type II diabetes (UKPDS 56). Clinical Science 2001; 101: 671–679.

19. Evans JMM, Wang J, Morris AD. Comparison of cardiovascular risk between patients with type 2 diabetes and those who had had a myocardial infarction: cross sectional and cohort studies. BMJ 2002; 324: 939–943.

20. Heart Protection Study Collaborative Group. MRC/BHF Heart Protection Study of cholesterol-lowering with simvastatin in 5963 people with diabetes: a randomised placebo-controlled trial. Lancet 2003; 361: 2005–2016.

21. Al-Delaimy WK, Willett WC, Manson JE, et al. Smoking and mortality among women with type 2 diabetes: The Nurses' Health Study cohort. Diabetes Care 2001; 24(12): 2043–2048.

22. Haire-Joshu D, Glasgow RE, Tibbs TL. Smoking and diabetes. Diabetes Care 1999; 22(11): 1887–1898.

23. CDC Diabetes Cost-effectiveness Group. Cost-effectiveness of intensive glycemic control, intensified hypertension control, and serum cholesterol level reduction for type 2 diabetes. JAMA 2002; 287(19): 2542–2551.

24. National Health Committee. Guidelines for smoking cessation (revised May 2002). Wellington: National Health Committee; 2002.

25. UK Prospective Diabetes Study Group. Tight blood pressure control and risk of macrovascular and microvascular complications in type 2 diabetes: UKPDS 38. BMJ 1998; 317(7160): 703–713.

26. Antithrombotic Trialists' Collaboration. Collaborative meta-analysis of randomised trials of antiplatelet therapy for prevention of death, myocardial infarction, and stroke in high risk patients. BMJ 2002; 324(7329): 71–86.

27. Sanmuganathan PS, Ghahramani P, Jackson PR, et al. Aspirin for primary prevention of coronary heart disease: safety and absolute benefit related to coronary risk derived from meta-analysis of randomised trials. Heart 2001; 85(3): 265–271.

28. Gaede P, Vedel P, Larsen N, et al. Multifactorial intervention and cardiovascular disease in patients with type 2 diabetes. New England Journal of Medicine 2003; 348(5): 383–393.

29. Wald NJ, Law MR. A strategy to reduce cardiovascular disease by more than 80%. BMJ 2003; 326(7404): 1419.

30. Trewby PN, Reddy AV, Trewby CS, et al. Are preventive drugs preventive enough? A study of patients' expectation of benefits from preventive drugs. Clinical Medicine 2002; 2(6): 527–533.

31. Vijan S, Hayward RA. Treatment of hypertension in type 2 diabetes mellitus: blood pressure goals, choice of agents, and setting priorities in diabetes care. Archives of Internal Medicine 2003; 138(7): 593–602.

32. Williams B, Poulter NR, Brown MJ, et al. British Hypertension Society guidelines for hypertension management 2004 (BHS-IV): summary. BMJ 2004; 328: 634–640.

33. ALLHAT Officers and Coordinators for the ALLHAT Collaborative Research Group. Major outcomes in high-risk hypertensive patients randomized to angiotensin-converting enzyme inhibitor

or calcium channel blocker vs diuretic: The Antihypertensive and Lipid-Lowering Treatment to Prevent Heart Attack Trial (ALLHAT). JAMA 2002; 288(23): 2981–2997.

34. Parving H, Lehnert H, Brochner-Mortensen J, et al. The effect of irbesartan on the development of diabetic nephropathy in patients with type 2 diabetes. New England Journal of Medicine 2001; 345(12): 870–878.

35. Brenner BM, Cooper ME, de Zeeuw D, et al. Effects of losartan on renal and cardiovascular outcomes in patients with type 2 diabetes and nephropathy. New England Journal of Medicine 2001; 345(12): 861–869.

36. Lewis EJ, Hunsicker LG, Clarke WR, et al. Renoprotective effect of the angiotensin-receptor antagonist irbesartan in patients with nephropathy due to type 2 diabetes. New England Journal of Medicine 2001; 345(12): 851–860.

37. Nakao N, Yoshimura A, Morita H, et al. Combination treatment of angiotensin-II receptor blocker and angiotensin-converting-enzyme inhibitor in non-diabetic renal disease (COOPERATE): a randomised controlled trial. Lancet 2003; 361(9352): 117–124.

38. Randomised trial of cholesterol lowering in 4444 patients with coronary heart disease: the Scandinavian Simvastatin Survival Study (4S). Lancet 1994; 344(8934): 1383–1389.

39. Shepherd J, Cobbe SM, Ford I. Prevention of coronary heart disease with pravastatin in men with hypercholesterolaemia (WOSCOPS). New England Journal of Medicine 1995; 333: 1301–1307.

40. MRC/BHF Heart Protection Study of cholesterol lowering with simvastatin in 20,536 high-risk individuals: a randomised placebo-controlled trial. Lancet 2002; 360(9326): 7–22.

41. Long-Term Intervention with Pravastatin in Ischaemic Disease (LIPID) Study Group. Prevention of cardiovascular events and death with pravastatin in patients with coronary heart disease and a broad range of initial cholesterol levels. New England Journal of Medicine 1998; 339(19): 1349–1357.

42. Effect of fenofibrate on progression of coronary-artery disease in type 2 diabetes: the Diabetes Atherosclerosis Intervention Study, a randomised study. Lancet 2001; 357(9260): 905–910.

43. Rubins HB, Robins SJ, Collins D. Gemfibrozil for the secondary prevention of coronary heart disease in men with low levels of high-density lipoprotein cholesterol. The Veterans Affairs High-Density Lipoprotein Cholesterol Intervention Study Group. New England Journal of Medicine 1999; 341: 410–418.

44. Yusuf S, Sleight P, Pogue J, et al. Effects of an angiotensin-converting-enzyme inhibitor, ramipril, on cardiovascular events in high-risk patients. The Heart Outcomes Prevention Evaluation Study Investigators. New England Journal of Medicine 2000; 342(3): 145–153.

45. Marre M, Lievre M, Chatellier G, et al. Effects of low dose ramipril on cardiovascular and renal outcomes in patients with type 2 diabetes and raised excretion of urinary albumin: randomised, double blind, placebo controlled trial (the DIABHYCAR study). BMJ 2004; 328: 495–499.

46. Dahlof B, Devereux RB, Kjeldsen SE, et al. Cardiovascular morbidity and mortality in the Losartan Intervention For Endpoint reduction in hypertension study (LIFE): a randomised trial against atenolol. Lancet 2002; 359(9311): 995–1003.

47. Law MR, Wald NJ. Risk factor thresholds: their existence under scrutiny. BMJ 2002; 324(7353): 1570–1576.

48. Malmberg K. Prospective randomized study of intensive insulin treatment on long term survival after acute myocardial infarction in patients with diabetes. DIGAMI (Diabetes Mellitus, Insulin Glucose Infusion in Acute Myocardial Infarction) Study Group. BMJ 1997; 314: 1512–1515.
49. Wald DS, Law M, Morris JK. Homocysteine and cardiovascular disease: evidence on causality from a meta-analysis. BMJ 2002; 325(7374): 1202.

## Chapter 14

1. Parving H. Initiation and progression of diabetic nephropathy. New England Journal of Medicine 1996; 335(22): 1682–1683.
2. Remuzzi G, Schieppati A, Ruggenenti P. Clinical practice. Nephropathy in patients with type 2 diabetes. New England Journal of Medicine 2002; 346(15): 1145 1151.
3. The Diabetes Control and Complications Trial/Epidemiology of Diabetes Interventions and Complications Research Group. Retinopathy and nephropathy in patients with type 1 diabetes four years after a trial of intensive therapy. New England Journal of Medicine 2000; 342(6): 381–389.
4. Simmons D, Schaumkel J, Cecil A, et al. High impact of nephropathy on five-year mortality rates among patients with Type 2 diabetes mellitus from a multi-ethnic population in New Zealand. Diabetic Medicine 1999; 16: 926–931.
5. Schmitz A, Vaeth M. Microalbuminuria: a major risk factor in non-insulin-dependent diabetes. A 10-year follow-up study of 503 patients. Diabetic Medicine 1988: 5: 126–134.
6. Hovind P, Tarnow L, Rossing K, et al. Decreasing incidence of severe diabetic microangiopathy in type 1 diabetes. Diabetes Care 2003; 26(4): 1258–1264.
7. Adler AI, Stevens RJ, Manley SE, et al. Development and progression of nephropathy in type 2 diabetes: The United Kingdom Prospective Diabetes Study (UKPDS 64). Kidney International 2003; 63(1): 225–232.
8. Lewis EJ, Hunsicker LG, Bain RP, et al. The effect of angiotensin-converting-enzyme inhibition on diabetic nephropathy. The Collaborative Study Group. New England Journal of Medicine 1993; 329: 1456–1462.
9. Lewis EJ, Hunsicker LG, Clarke WR, et al. Renoprotective effect of the angiotensin-receptor antagonist irbesartan in patients with nephropathy due to type 2 diabetes. New England Journal of Medicine 2001; 345(12): 851–860.
10. Brenner BM, Cooper ME, de Zeeuw D, et al. Effects of losartan on renal and cardiovascular outcomes in patients with type 2 diabetes and nephropathy. New England Journal of Medicine 2001; 345(12): 861–869.
11. Nakao N, Yoshimura A, Morita H, et al. Combination treatment of angiotensin-II receptor blocker and angiotensin-converting-enzyme inhibitor in non-diabetic renal disease (COOPERATE): a randomised controlled trial. Lancet 2003; 361(9352): 117–124.
12. Muhlhauser I, Bender R, Bott U, et al. Cigarette smoking and progression of retinopathy and nephropathy in type 1 diabetes. Diabetic Medicine 1996; 13(6): 536–543.
13. Parving H, Lehnert H, Brochner-Mortensen J, et al. The effect of irbesartan on the development of diabetic nephropathy in patients with type 2 diabetes. New England Journal of Medicine 2001; 345(12): 870–878.
14. Mathiesen ER, Hommel E, Hansen HP, et al. Randomised controlled trial of long term efficacy of captopril on preservation of kidney function in

normotensive patients with insulin dependent diabetes and microalbuminuria. BMJ 1999; 319(7201): 24–25.

15. Gaede P, Vedel P, Larsen N, et al. Multifactorial intervention and cardiovascular disease in patients with type 2 diabetes. New England Journal of Medicine 2003; 348(5): 383–393.

16. Marshall SM. Blood pressure control, microalbuminuria and cardiovascular risk in Type 2 diabetes mellitus. Diabetic Medicine 1999; 16(5): 358–372.

17. Mogensen CE. Microalbuminuria, blood pressure and diabetic renal disease: origin and development of ideas. Diabetologia 1999; 42(3): 263–285.

18. MacIsaac RJ, Smith TJ, Tsalamandris C, et al. Nonalbuminuric renal insufficiency in type 2 diabetes. Diabetes Care 2004; 27: 195–200.

## Chapter 15

1. Moss SE, Klein R, Klein BEK. The incidence of vision loss in a diabetic population. Ophthalmology 1988; 95: 1340–1348.

2. Klein R, Klein BE, Moss SE, et al. The Wisconsin epidemiologic study of diabetic retinopathy II. Prevalence and risk of diabetic retinopathy when age at diagnosis is less than 30 years. Archives of Ophthalmology 1984; 102: 520–526.

3. Klein R, Klein BE, Moss SE, et al. The Wisconsin epidemiologic study of diabetic retinopathy III. Prevalence and risk of diabetic retinopathy when age at diagnosis is 30 or more years. Archives of Ophthalmology 1984; 102: 527–532.

4. Davis MD, Norton EWD, Myers FL. The Airlie classification of diabetic retinopathy. In: Goldberg MF, Fine SL (eds) Symposium on the Treatment of Diabetic Retinopathy, Airlie House, Warrenton, Virginia: US Department of Health, Education and Welfare; 1968; p 7–37.

5. Stratton IM, Kohner EM, Aldington SJ, et al. UKPDS 50: risk factors for incidence and progression of retinopathy in Type II diabetes over 6 years from diagnosis. Diabetologia 2001;44(2):156–163.

6. Porta M, Sjoelie AK, Chaturvedi N, et al. Risk factors for progression to proliferative diabetic retinopathy in the EURODIAB Prospective Complications Study. Diabetologia 2001; 44: 2203–2209.

7. The effect of intensive treatment of diabetes on the development and progression of long-term complications in insulin-dependent diabetes mellitus. The Diabetes Control and Complications Trial Research Group. New England Journal of Medicine 1993; 329(14): 977–986.

8. UK Prospective Diabetes Study (UKPDS) Group. Intensive blood-glucose control with sulphonylureas or insulin compared with conventional treatment and risk of complications in patients with type 2 diabetes (UKPDS 33). Lancet 1998; 352: 837–853.

9. UK Prospective Diabetes Study Group. Tight blood pressure control and risk of macrovascular and microvascular complications in type 2 diabetes: UKPDS 38. BMJ 1998; 317(7160): 703–713.

10. Bergerhoff K, Clar C, Richter B. Aspirin in diabetic retinopathy. A systematic review. Endocrinology and Metabolism Clinics of North America 2002; 31: 779–793.

11. Hutchinson A, McIntosh A, Peters J, et al. Effectiveness of screening and monitoring tests for diabetic retinopathy – a systematic review. Diabetic Medicine 2000; 17(7): 495–506.

12. Hutchinson A, McIntosh A, Peters J, et al. Clinical guidelines and evidence review for Type 2 diabetes. Diabetic retinopathy: early management and screening. Sheffield: ScHARR, University of Sheffield; 2001.

13. Vijan S, Hofer TP, Hayward RA. Cost–utility analysis of screening intervals for diabetic retinopathy in patients with type 2 diabetes mellitus. JAMA 2000; 283(7): 889–896.
14. Younis N, Broadbent D, Vora J, et al. Incidence of sight-threatening retinopathy in patients with type 2 diabetes in the Liverpool Diabetic Eye Study: a cohort study. Lancet. 2003; 361(9353): 195–200.
15. Early worsening of diabetic retinopathy in the Diabetes Control and Complications Trial. Archives of Ophthalmology 1998; 116(7): 874–886.
16. Kohner E. Photocoagulation in the prevention of blindness due to diabetic retinopathy: a review. Journal of the Royal Society of Medicine 1984; 77(3): 227–233.
17. Photocoagulation for diabetic macular edema. Early Treatment Diabetic Retinopathy Study report number 1. Early Treatment Diabetic Retinopathy Study research group. Archives of Ophthalmology 1985; 103(12): 1796–1806.
18. Chaturvedi N, Sjolie AK, Stephenson JM, et al. Effect of lisinopril on progression of retinopathy in normotensive people with type 1 diabetes. The EUCLID Study Group. EURODIAB Controlled Trial of Lisinopril in Insulin-Dependent Diabetes Mellitus. Lancet 1998; 351(9095): 28–31.

## Chapter 16

1. Dejgaard A. Pathophysiology and treatment of diabetic neuropathy. Diabetic Medicine 1998; 15(2): 97–112.
2. Walter DP, Gatling W, Mullee MA, et al. The prevalence of diabetic distal sensory neuropathy in an English community. Diabetic Medicine 1992; 9: 349–353.
3. Young MJ, Boulton AJM, Macleod AF, et al. A multicentre study of the prevalence of diabetic peripheral neuropathy in the United Kingdom hospital clinic population. Diabetologia 1993; 36: 150–154.
4. The Diabetes Control and Complications Trial Research Group. The effect of intensive diabetes therapy on the development and progression of neuropathy. Annals of Internal Medicine 1995; 122(8): 561–568.
5. Cameron NE, Eaton SE, Cotter MA, et al. Vascular factors and metabolic interactions in the pathogenesis of diabetic neuropathy. Diabetologia 2001; 44(11): 1973–1988.
6. Boulton AJM, Gries FA, Jervell JA. Guidelines for the diagnosis and outpatient management of diabetic peripheral neuropathy. Diabetic Medicine 1998; 15: 508–514.
7. Benbow SJ, Cossins L, MacFarlane IA. Painful diabetic neuropathy. Diabetic Medicine 1999; 16(8): 632–644.
8. Backonja M, Beydoun A, Edwards KR, et al. Gabapentin for the symptomatic treatment of painful neuropathy in patients with diabetes mellitus: a randomized controlled trial. JAMA 1998; 280(21): 1831–1836.
9. Boulton AJ. Lowering the risk of neuropathy, foot ulcers and amputations. Diabetic Medicine 1998; 15(Suppl 4): S57–59.
10. Vinik AI, Maser RE, Mitchell BD, et al. Diabetic autonomic neuropathy. Diabetes Care 2003; 26(5): 1553–1579.

## Chapter 17

1. Mason J, O'Keeffe C, Hutchinson A, et al. A systematic review of foot ulcer in patients with Type 2 diabetes mellitus. II: treatment. Diabetic Medicine 1999; 16(11): 889–909.
2. Mason J, O'Keeffe C, McIntosh A, et al. A systematic review of foot ulcer in

patients with Type 2 diabetes mellitus. I: prevention. Diabetic Medicine 1999; 16(10): 801–812.

3. Watkins PJ. ABC of diabetes: the diabetic foot. BMJ 2003; 326(7396): 977–979.

4. Abbott CA, Carrington AL, Ashe H, et al. The North-West Diabetes Foot Care Study: incidence of, and risk factors for, new diabetic foot ulceration in a community-based patient cohort. Diabetic Medicine 2002; 19: 377–384.

5. Tapp RJ, Shaw JE, de Courten MP, et al. Foot complications in Type 2 diabetes: an Australian population-based study. Diabetic Medicine 2003; 20(2): 105–113.

6. Hutchinson A, McIntosh A, Feder G, et al. Clinical guidelines and evidence review for Type 2 diabetes: prevention and management of foot problems. London: Royal College of General Practitioners; 2000.

7. Boulton AJ. Lowering the risk of neuropathy, foot ulcers and amputations. Diabetic Medicine 1998; 15(Suppl 4): S57–59.

8. A strategy for arterial risk assessment and management in type 2 (non-insulin-dependent) diabetes mellitus. European Arterial Risk Policy Group on behalf of the International Diabetes Federation European Region. Diabetic Medicine 1997; 14(7): 611–621.

9. Connor H. Diabetic foot disease – where is the evidence? Diabetic Medicine 1999; 16(10): 799–800.

10. Edmonds ME, Blundell MP, Morris ME, et al. Improved survival of the diabetic foot: the role of a specialized foot clinic. QJM 1986; 232: 763–771.

11. Reiber GE, Smith DG, Wallace C, et al. Effect of therapeutic footwear on foot reulceration in patients with diabetes: a randomized controlled trial. JAMA 2002; 287(19): 2552–2558.

12. Jeffcoate W, Lima J, Nobrega L. The Charcot foot. Diabetic Medicine 2000; 17(4): 253–258.

13. Rajbhandari SM, Jenkins RC, Davies C, et al. Charcot neuroarthropathy in diabetes mellitus. Diabetologia 2002; 45(8): 1085–1096.

14. Adler AI, Boyko EJ, Ahroni JH, et al. Lower-extremity amputation in diabetes. The independent effects of peripheral vascular disease, sensory neuropathy, and foot ulcers. Diabetes Care 1999; 22: 1029–1042.

## Chapter 18

1. Angulo P. Nonalcoholic fatty liver disease. New England Journal of Medicine 2002; 346(16): 1221–1231.

2. Clark JM, Diehl AM. Nonalcoholic fatty liver disease: an underrecognized cause of cryptogenic cirrhosis. JAMA 2003; 289(22): 3000–3004.

3. Shah BR, Hux JE. Quantifying the risk of infectious diseases for people with diabetes. Diabetes Care 2003; 26(2): 510–513.

4. Joshi N, Caputo GM, Weitekamp MR, et al. Infections in patients with diabetes mellitus. New England Journal of Medicine 1999; 341(25): 1906–1912.

5. Holmes GK. Coeliac disease and Type 1 diabetes mellitus – the case for screening. Diabetic Medicine 2001; 18(3): 169–177.

6. Bloomgarden ZT. Diabetes issues in women and children: polycystic ovary syndrome. Diabetes Care 2003; 26(8): 2457–2463.

7. Calle EE, Rodriguez C, Walker-Thurmond K, et al. Overweight, obesity, and mortality from cancer in a prospectively studied cohort of U.S. adults. New England Journal of Medicine 2003; 348(17): 1625–1638.

## Further reading

Any selection of books on diabetes is personal and dependent upon the need, but we believe the following few have met the test of time and fulfil particular needs. Be sure you are using the latest edition!

Day JL. Living with diabetes. The Diabetes UK guide for those treated with diet and tablets. Chichester: Wiley, 2001.

Day JL. Living with diabetes. The Diabetes UK guide for those treated with insulin. Chichester: Wiley, 2002.

Gill GV, Pickup JC, Williams G (eds) Difficult diabetes. Oxford: Blackwell, 2001.

Mackinnon M. Providing diabetes care in general practice: a practical guide for the primary care team, 4th edn. London: Class Publishing, 2002.

Watkins PJ. An ABC of diabetes, 5th edn. London: BMJ Publishing, 2003.

Williams R (ed). The evidence base for diabetes care. Chichester: Wiley, 2002.

For details of other patient books go to *www.diabetes.co.uk/HTM/GIFTS/books2. htm.*

# GLOSSARY
## Studies and trials in diabetes

**4S** – Scandinavian Simvastatin Survival Study

**ABCD** – Appropriate Blood Pressure Control in Diabetes [Trial]

**ALLHAT** – Antihypertensive and Lipid Lowering to prevent Heart Attack Trial

**ASPEN** – Prevention of CHD Endpoints in Patients with Non-Insulin-Dependent Diabetes Mellitus [Study]

**AUSDIAB** – Australian Diabetes, Obesity and Lifestyle Study

**CARDS** – Collaborative Atorvastatin Diabetes Study

**CARE** – Cholesterol and Recurrent Events [Study]

**DAIS** – Diabetes Atherosclerosis Intervention Study

**DAWN** – Diabetes, Attitudes, Wishes and Needs [Study]

**DCCT** – Diabetes Control and Complications Trial

**DIGAMI** – Diabetes mellitus, Insulin Glucose infusion in Acute Myocardial Infarction [Study]

**DPP** – Diabetes Prevention Program [Trial]

**FIELD** – Fenofibrate Intervention and Event Lowering in Diabetes [Study]

**HERS** – Heart and Estrogen/Progestin Replacement Study

**HHS** – Helsinki Heart Study

**HIT** – HDL Intervention Trial

**HOPE** – Heart Outcomes Prevention Evaluation [Study]

**HOT** – Hypertension Optimisation Trial

**HPS** – Heart Protection Study

**IDNT** – International Diabetic Nephropathy Trial

**Kumamoto** – Kumamoto study of improved control in type 2 diabetes

**LIFE** – Losartan Intervention For Endpoint reduction in hypertension [study]

**LIPID** – Long-term Intervention with Pravastatin in Ischaemic Disease [Study]

**MRFIT** – Multiple Risk Factor Intervention Trial

**NCEP** – National Cholesterol Education Program (US)

**NZGG** – New Zealand Guidelines Group

**SHEP** – Systolic Hypertension in the Elderly Program

**SIGN** – Scottish Intercollegiate Guidelines Network

**STOP-NIDDM** – acarbose trial in prevention of type 2 diabetes

**SystEur** – Systolic Hypertension in Europe [Trial]

**UKPDS** – United Kingdom Prospective Diabetes Study

**WHI** – Women's Health Initiative [Study]

**WOSCOPS** – West of Scotland Coronary Prevention Study

# LIST OF PATIENT QUESTIONS

# INDEX

Note:

Abbreviations

IFG - impaired fasting glucose

IGT - impaired glucose tolerance

OHA - oral hypoglycaemic agent

As diabetes mellitus is the subject of this book, all index entries refer to diabetes unless otherwise indicated.

Entries have been kept to a minimum under 'diabetes' or 'diabetic' and readers are advised to seek more specific entries.

Page numbers in **bold** refer to figures/tables/boxes.

## A

Abciximab, 220

Abscesses, 284

Absolute risk, 199, **199**

Acanthosis nigricans, 284

Acarbose, **80**, 86

actions, 79

side effects and contraindications, **80**

STOP-NIDDM study, 14

ACE inhibitors

hypertension treatment, 210, **211**, 212, 213

microalbuminuria treatment, 40, 235

in nephropathy treatment, 233, **234**

pre-conception counselling, 181

pros and cons in diabetes, 211

retinopathy treatment, 256

risks, in diabetic renal disease, 235

routine use, evidence for, 217

side effects, 211, 235

Acipimox, 217

Acromegaly, 48

Actrapid, self-testing of blood glucose results, **166**

Addison's disease, **286**

Adherence to medication, poor *see* Non-compliance with medication

Adolescents, type 2 diabetes prevalence, 21

Aetiology of diabetes *see* Pathophysiology/aetiology of diabetes

Age

neuropathy prevalence, **258**, 258–259

pregnancy complications in diabetes, 187–188

type 2 diabetes prevalence, 19, **20**, 20–21

weight gain with, 68

Age of onset, type 1 *vs* type 2 diabetes, **50**

Air travel, 174

Albumin:creatinine ratio (ACR), 227, 236, **236**

Alcohol, intake

choice (wine *vs* beer), 76

driving avoidance, 76

health benefits, 75

healthy drinking limits, 75

high, 50, 51

nocturnal hypoglycaemia, 137

painful neuropathy, 261

poorly controlled diabetes, 125

recommendations, 59

Alcoholic liver disease, 282

Allergy, insulin, 106

ALLHAT study, 210, 211, 212, 217

Alpha (α)-cells, glucagon secretion, 3

Alpha-glucosidase inhibitor *see* Acarbose

Alternative therapies, 173

American Diabetes Association, 295

Amfebutamone (Zyban), 206

Amitriptyline, neuropathic pain relief, 263, 265

Amputation, 39, 270, 273

frequency and prevention, 279

risk factors, 272

Amyotrophy, femoral, 258, 260, 263

Analgesics, neuropathic pain relief, 263, 265

Angina, 205

Angioplasty, 220, 275

Angiotensin 2 receptor antagonists, 212–213, 217

microalbuminuria treatment, 235

in nephropathy treatment, 233

retinopathy treatment, 256

risks, in diabetic renal disease, 235

side effects, 235

Angiotensin-converting enzyme (ACE) inhibitors *see* ACE inhibitors

Ankle/brachial pressure ratio, 273

Ankle reflexes, 262

Annual reviews, 155

protocol, **155–156**

Anticonvulsants, 264

Antidepressants, 168

neuropathic pain management, 263

during weight loss, 69

Anti-gliadin antibodies, 286

## B

# D

# E

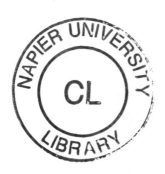